THE ANTIOXIDANT VITAMIN COUNTER

Annette B. Natow, Ph.D., R.D., and Jo-Ann Heslin, M.A., R.D.

POCKET BOOKS

New York London Toronto Sydney Tokyo Singapore

An *Original* Publication of POCKET BOOKS

POCKET BOOKS, a division of Simon & Schuster Inc.
1230 Avenue of the Americas, New York, NY 10020

ISBN: 0-671-78320-3

First Pocket Books printing March 1994

10 9 8 7 6 5 4

POCKET and colophon are registered trademarks of Simon & Schuster Inc.

Cover design by Tom McKeveny

inted in the U.S.A.

To our families, who support us through every
project: Harry, Allen, Irene, Sarah, Meryl, Laura,
Marty, George, Emily, Steven, Joe,
Kristen and Karen.

ACKNOWLEDGMENTS

Without the tireless cooperation of Steven and Stephen, *The Antioxidant Vitamin Counter* would never have been completed. Our thanks to Dr. Irene E. Rosenberg and Alma Flaumenhaft for reviewing the material. A special thanks to our editor, Rebecca Todd, and our agent, Nancy Trichter.

————————

"Certain foods have already begun to stand out, however, as rich and economical sources of these newer dietary essentials."

"To be rich in the A vitamin, its leaves must be really green, not white."

"Fresh fruits . . . are particularly valuable for their contribution."

MARY SWARTZ ROSE, PH. D.
Feeding the Family
The Macmillan Company, 1919

CONTENTS

SOURCES OF DATA

Values in this counter have been obtained from the Composition of Foods, United States Department of Agriculture, Agricultural Handbooks: No. 8-1, Dairy and Egg Products; No. 8-2, Spices and Herbs; No. 8-3, Baby Foods; No. 8-4, Fats and Oils; No. 8-5, Poultry Products; No. 8-6, Soups, Sauces and Gravies; No. 8-7, Sausages and Luncheon Meats; No. 8-8, Breakfast Cereals; No. 8-9 Fruit and Fruit Juices; No. 8-10, Pork Products; No. 8-11, Vegetables and Vegetable Products; No. 8-12, Nut and Seed Products; No. 8-13, Beef Products; No. 8-14, Beverages; No. 8-15, Finfish and Shellfish Products; No. 8-16, Legumes and Legume Products; No. 8-17, Lamb, Veal and Game Products; No. 8-18, Baked Products; No. 8-19, Snacks and Sweets; No. 8-20, Cereal Grains and Pasta; No. 8-21, Fast Foods; Supplements 1989, 1990, 1991.

Nutritive Value of Foods, United States Department of Agriculture, Home and Garden Bulletin No. 72.

J. Davies and J. Dickerson, *Nutrient Content of Food Portions* (Cambridge, UK: The Royal Society of Chemistry, 1991).

G. A. Leveille, M. E. Zabik, K. J. Morgan, *Nutrients in Foods* (Cambridge, MA: The Nutrition Guild, 1983).

Souci, Fachmann, Kraut, *Food Composition and Nutri-*

tion Tables (Stuttgart: Wissenschaftliche Verlagsgesellschaft MbH, 1989).

Information from food labels, manufacturers and processors. The values are based on research conducted through 1993. Manufacturers' ingredients are subject to change, so current values may vary from those listed in this book.

INTRODUCTION

NATURAL ENEMIES, NATURAL PROTECTORS

Free radicals—the body's natural enemies—are made every day in the body and are very damaging to normal molecules in healthy cells that are near them.

Antioxidants—the body's natural protectors—are made every day in the body and every day we eat antioxidant-rich foods, containing vitamins A, C, and E, that protect against free radicals.

The goal is to have a balance between the natural enemies and the natural protectors. **Many of us fall short of this goal, putting us at risk for heart disease, cancer, reduced immunity and other serious illness.**

This book lists the antioxidant vitamin content of more than 7,000 foods. For the first time, information about anti-oxidant values is at your fingertips. Now you will find it easy to follow a healthy diet. Before *The Antioxidant Vitamin Counter* it was impossible to compare so many foods at one time.

THE RADICAL CONNECTION

What do sunlight, exercise, air pollution, cigarettes, car exhaust, ozone, x-rays, chemotherapy and everyday living have in common?

They all produce "free radicals" in the healthy body. Researchers believe the damage by free radicals can cause: *aging, heart disease, cancer, reduced immune function, cataracts, Parkinson's disease, arthritis, and emphysema.*

Natural Enemies
FREE RADICALS

What are free radicals?

Dangerous hyperactive molecules.

Natural Protectors
ANTIOXIDANTS

What are antioxidants?

Substances both made in the body plus the vitamins C, E, and beta-carotene (the chemical parent to vitamin A) that block the damage from free radicals.

What do they do?

Free radicals rampage around the body damaging cells, disrupting their genetic blueprint and their ability to work.

What do they do?

Antioxidants function as the body's police force, collaring and hauling away dangerous free radicals.

What happens next?

When free radicals are left unchecked, the damage they do to body cells sets the stage for cancer, heart disease, birth defects, reduced immune function and premature aging.

What happens next?

Antioxidants prevent damage from free radicals and let the body's natural healing process work—promoting good health, slowing down aging and keeping cells healthy.

THE PRICE WE PAY FOR LIVING

We all know that oxygen is necessary for life. By combining oxygen with the foods we eat—oxidizing it—the body generates the energy we need to live. While using oxygen to produce energy is very efficient, it carries a price—the production of unstable oxygen byproducts called "free radicals," which are oxygen atoms that have been stripped of one electron. These hyperactive molecules readily attack molecules in our healthy cells, damaging them and forming more free radicals in a chain reaction. These damaged body cells no longer work normally and may result in tumors, cataracts, decreased immunity and clogged arteries. For example, evidence is accumulating that only after cholesterol has been oxidized by free radicals does it stick to the artery walls, narrowing them and setting the stage for blockage and heart attack.

"Through free radical reactions in our body, it's as though we're being irradiated at low levels all the time. They grind us down."

—Lester Packer, biochemist,
University of California, Berkeley

The natural protectors—antioxidants—stop the damage from free radicals. Antioxidant vitamins C, E and the plant form of vitamin A are among the most important antioxidants. For example, when vitamin E is on the surface of the lungs, it mops up free radicals and stops them from attacking lung cells and damaging them.

"The evidence is really mounting that antioxidants really protect against cardiovascular events such as heart attacks and strokes," said Dr. Joann Manson of Harvard Medical School. In her study on women and strokes, based on female nurses across the United States, she found that eating antioxidant-rich spinach and carrots were protective against strokes.

At a recent medical meeting, a survey showed that more than half of the nutrition researchers present were taking antioxidant vitamins daily. *The Medical Tribune,* a bimonthly newspaper with over 130,000 physician subscribers, recently conducted a poll on physicians' use of vitamin E. Hundreds of responders reported that they use vitamin E themselves and recommend it to patients for cardiovascular disease, high blood cholesterol, high blood pressure, heart valve disease, and as a general antioxidant for good health. Doses range from 100 to 800 IU a day.

The message is clear. It's time for us all to eat more fruits and vegetables to increase our intake of the protective antioxidants.

"I'm ashamed to do it (take a supplement) because of my attitude toward taking vitamins. But an explosion of studies shows that vitamin E is a possible preventative for heart disease, cancer and dozens of other disorders."

—Dr. Max Horwitt, Professor Emeritus,
St. Louis University School of Medicine

WHY FOOD IS BETTER THAN PILLS

"Eat your carrots, eat your kale, eat your broccoli. The supplements should be on top of a terrific diet."

—Dr. Michael Jacobson, Executive Director,
Center for Science in the Public Interest

What contains fiber, vitamins, minerals, phytochemicals, pigments, energy and other valuable substances?—*FOOD.* That's why a supplement can never substitute for eating. Supplements are a valuable addition to eating well. But *eating well* is the foundation for good health and boosts your antioxidant intake.

EATING ANTIOXIDANTS

The evidence mounts daily. The more antioxidant-rich foods you eat, the healthier you are. Most of us don't get enough of these important compounds. Public health messages from many sources recommend five or more fruits and vegetables a day. The average American eats one! Less than 10 percent are following the recommendation. The rest of us need to do better.

- Eighty percent of adults do not eat fruit and vegetables rich in vitamin A.
- Seventy-two percent of adults do not eat fruits and vegetables rich in vitamin C.
- Most Americans do not meet the daily recommendation for vitamin E.

How much is enough? Probably far more than you are eating.
Your daily antioxidant goal should be:

Vitamin	Suggested Daily Intake	Intake From Food
A	5,000 IU	4,000 IU from plant sources
C	250–500 MG	250 MG
E	100–200 IU	15–25 IU

This suggested daily antioxidant intake is high. You may not be able to get it all from food. Experts feel that you can eat enough antioxidant-rich food to meet the goal for vitamins A and C, but it's tougher for vitamin E.

"I doubt that you can get enough vitamin E through even a healthy diet, unless you want to drink too much oil, salad dressing, or other fatty foods like that. But vitamin C and beta-carotene you probably can get. The problem, of course, is that people don't."

—Dr. Jeffrey B. Blumberg, Associate Director, U.S. Department of Agriculture's Human Nutrition Research Center on Aging at Tufts University

Start by choosing vitamin E–rich foods.

GOOD: Dark green vegetables, fruits, whole grains
BETTER: Vegetables oils, nuts, seeds
BEST: Wheat germ

Consider making up the difference with a vitamin E supplement. A supplement of 100 IU of E a day is the perfect complement to a good diet. You may not be able to find vitamin E supplements in 100 IU doses. The most usual amounts are 200, 400 or 1000 IU. Don't be concerned about this. You don't have to take a supplement daily to benefit from it. You can take a 200 IU supplement every other day, the 400 IU twice a week, or the 1000 IU supplement once a week.

To make your diet antioxidant-rich try the following.

MORNING
- Drink juice rich in vitamin C (grapefruit, tomato, orange)
- Add sliced strawberries, raspberries or blueberries to cereal
- Have a bowl of fresh cantaloupe, peaches, persimmons, mango, papaya, watermelon, strawberries or apricots
- Add wheat germ to yogurt, cereal, pancakes or waffles
- Choose oatmeal and other whole grain cereals

LUNCH
- Have a green leafy salad or soup with carrots
- Top yogurt with wheat germ, sunflower seeds or nuts
- Eat fruit for dessert
- Add lettuce, tomato or grated carrots to a sandwich
- Choose rye and other whole grain breads

SNACK
- Nibble on dried papaya, apricots or peaches
- Use fruit juice as a between-meal refresher
- Eat raw carrots, broccoli or red and green peppers
- Choose sorbet or a fresh fruit shake at the juice bar

DINNER
- Serve a vegetable and salad every night
- Add grated carrot, chickpeas and soybeans to salads
- Have broccoli, cabbage, cauliflower and Brussels sprouts often
- Add vegetables to mixed dishes like pasta or casseroles
- Bake sweet potatoes or yams rather than white potatoes
- Choose cooked green or winter squash regularly
- Eat the parsley garnish
- Use pureed fruit sauces (plums, peach, apricots, prune) to garnish meats
- Top plain cakes with fresh fruit in season
- Top frozen yogurt with wheat germ and nuts
- Have a fruit salad as an appetizer or dessert

Other Bonuses

Many foods provide benefits beyond the obvious. Wheat bran, rice and red wine are good sources of many different antioxidants in addition to the antioxidant vitamins A, C, and E. Yogurt with active (live) cultures increases the production of gamma interferon, a substance that improves immune function. Gamma interferon may prevent viral infections, especially upper respiratory ones. Yogurt may also reduce food allergy symptoms. Carrots, green onions, kale, broccoli, cauliflower and Brussels sprouts contain sulforaphanes, powerful anti-cancer compounds. Preliminary evidence shows that tea, especially green tea, inhibits some cancers. Green tea contains several polyphenols, components that seem to protect cells from turning cancerous. Green tea and the regular black tea most of us drink come from the same plant. Black teas—such as orange pekoe, Earl Grey, English breakfast—are fermented. Green teas are simply picked and dried. Black tea retains some of its antioxidant properties but green tea has much more. Obviously much more research is needed before a pill can substitute for food.

A CLOSER LOOK AT ANTIOXIDANT VITAMIN A

THE PLANT FORM OF VITAMIN A

Vitamin A is found in foods in two different forms. In the plant form, it is found as carotenoids, color pigments which are the chemical parents of active vitamin A—the form used by the body. As needed, carotenoids are changed in the body into active vitamin A. Active vitamin A is also called preformed vitamin A, found in animal foods like milk, butter, eggs and meat. While carotenoids (plant sources) are anti-oxidants, preformed vitamin A is not. Once carotenoids are changed to active vitamin A, they no longer work as antioxidants.

Carotenoids, the antioxidant form of vitamin A, are part of a family of over 500 red and yellow pigments. About 50 of these can be changed to vitamin A in the body and, after conversion, they function as the vitamin promoting growth, vision and bone development.

A relation has been found between blood levels of vitamin A and the degree of recovery in stroke patients. A study done in Belgium found that stroke patients with high serum levels of vitamin A were more likely to have a complete recovery within the first twenty-four hours, a lower death rate and a better outcome as assessed by standard scales of neurological functioning.

Vitamin A used to be called the anti-infective vitamin because of its effect on skin (epithelial) cells. These cells make up skin and mucus membranes, the body's major barriers against invasion. This is the body's first line of defense against disease and infection.

Carotenoids, in high doses, enhance the body's immune function. Beta-carotene, the most studied carotenoid, is an antioxidant, and some other carotenoids act as antioxidants too. Carotenoids prevent damage by free radicals. They carry out these activities without being converted to vitamin A.

Beta-carotene has been studied more than the other carotenoids and has been shown to protect the body in many ways. But this doesn't mean that other carotenoids are not beneficial too. In fact, because different carotenoids are often found together in plant foods, it's not always certain exactly which one is providing the protection. It really doesn't matter because when you eat vegetables and fruits you get an assortment of carotenoids.

A study showed that giving beta-carotene to young men protected their immune system from the effects of ultraviolet light. Exposure to ultraviolet light from the sun and tanning salons has been shown to suppress immune functions. Sunscreens mainly protect the skin from the effects of one kind of ultraviolet light, UV-B radiation. Most sunscreens do not protect against UV-A, which damages the immune system. Beta-carotene protects the immune system against the effects of UV-A. When you are exposed to ultraviolet light, the requirement for beta-carotene goes up.

In another study when healthy, elderly people took beta-carotene every day for two months the immune system's beneficial killer cells were increased.

A preliminary study at the Oregon Health Sciences University in Portland has shown that beta-carotene might be helpful for HIV-infected people. When researchers gave twenty-one people infected with AIDS-causing HIV virus large doses of beta-carotene every day for four weeks their immune response improved.

Taking beta-carotene is good for the heart too. In the ongoing Harvard Physicians Health Study, a group of men who had experienced heart disease and chest pain (angina) experienced a dramatic reduction in heart attacks and other heart problems after taking beta-carotene every other day. Higher levels of beta-carotene in the blood were protective against heart attacks. Data from this group also show that the risk for heart disease of current and former smokers was lower where dietary intake of carotene was higher.

Eating plenty of carrots and spinach can lower a woman's risk of stroke, according to a new study presented at the 1993 American Heart Association Conference on Cardiovascular Disease and Epidemiology and Prevention. When studying over 87,000 female nurses, researchers found that those who ate five or more servings of carrots a week were two thirds less likely to have a stroke than those who ate one serving or less a month. Eating spinach also protected against stroke, but not as much as carrots.

Free radicals, the body's natural enemies, play a major role in causing cancer. As an antioxidant, beta-carotene can block the action of free radicals or repair the damage they cause. Many studies show that eating fruits and vegetables rich in beta-carotene reduced the risk of certain cancers. This was true of lung cancer even among people who smoked. In almost all studies, low intake of fruits and vegetables are consistently associated with a higher risk of lung cancer. There is evidence of a protective effect against cancers of the larynx, mouth, cervix, pancreas, stomach, esophagus, colon, and rectum when lots of fruits and vegetables are eaten.

Studies show that women who have cervical dysplasia (a precancerous condition), or cancer of the cervix, have lower levels of beta-carotene in their blood when compared to women who do not have cancer. The lower the blood level of beta-carotene the worse the condition.

When you eat more fruits and vegetables to get more beta-carotene, you not only increase your intake of the other antioxidants—C and E—you also get other protective substances that have not yet been fully studied. That is why vitamin supplements aren't as valuable as getting antioxidants through food.

". . . it is impossible to be confident that a particular factor is the effective agent . . . nature does not package a single nutrient in a particular food . . . the nutrient that is reported or reviewed reflects the interest of the investigator or reviewer . . . it is clear that nutrients act together, with optimal levels of several being required for optimal protection . . . the search for . . . a 'magic bullet' nutrient has led to insufficient appreciation of the strength and consistency of the evidence that fruits and vegetables themselves have an important protective effect against a very wide range of human cancers."

"Fruit, Vegetables, and Cancer Prevention: A Review of the Epidemiological Evidence," Gladys Block, School of Public Health, University of California, Berkeley

How much vitamin A do I need?

The new National Labeling and Education Act (NLEA) recommends a daily intake of 5000 IU as the Daily Value (DV) for food labels. Four thousand of the 5,000 IU recommended daily should come from plant sources of vitamin A—dark green, leafy vegetables like spinach and romaine lettuce, and yellow and orange vegetables and fruits like cantaloupe, carrots, and sweet potatoes.

Because of the overwhelming evidence showing that the antioxidant properties of beta-carotene and other carotenoids are important in maintaining health and the function of the immune system, it may be time to look at the recommendation in a new way. We need larger amounts of the plant form of vitamin A than many of us are getting in our usual diets. In fact, some of us, particularly those who are frequent fast-food eaters, may need to use vitamin supplements along with making better food choices whenever possible.

The National Research Council, the United States Department of Agriculture and the American Cancer Society recommend eating five or more servings of fruits and vegetables daily. Less than 10 percent of Americans eat that amount. It is important for everyone to eat more fruits and vegetables.

Can you have too much vitamin A or carotenoids?

It's impossible to overdose on the plant form of vitamin A, but it is possible to consume dangerously high levels of preformed vitamin A from animal foods or vitamin supplements. While it is hard to do this with food, you could do it by taking too many supplements. No one should take more than 10,000 IU of vitamin A a day. That is twice the Recommended Daily Allowance (RDA), which is 5,000 IU.

Ten to fifteen times the RDA for vitamin A may be poisonous. It can cause headache, nausea, double vision and chronic poisoning leading to liver damage, hair loss and bone problems. This happens when all the normal places vitamin A works in the body are saturated and the free vitamin A attacks the cells. Too much vitamin A can cause birth defects when too much is taken during pregnancy.

Because the plant forms of vitamin A, the carotenoids, cannot be changed very efficiently to vitamin A, excess amounts are not poisonous. Instead they are stored in body fat as carotene. Carotenes are yellow and can accumulate under the skin causing it to turn yellow.

MEASURING VITAMIN A

Pre-formed Vitamin A

Vitamin A is found in its active form in animal foods like liver, cod and halibut liver oils, milk, butter and eggs. You will often see it measured in IU, a measure of the vitamin activity. IU are often determined by feeding some of the vitamin to a vitamin-deprived animal and then measuring its growth. The newer way of measuring vitamin A activity is as RE (retinol equivalents). You can convert IU to RE by simple multiplication: 1 RE = 3.33 IU.

Carotenoids

Plant forms of vitamin A, carotenoids, are also measured in IU and RE and also in milligrams (mg). Again some multiplication is needed to convert one measurement to another: 1 RE = 10.00 IU.

To change beta-carotenes from IU to milligrams and the other way around:

        For IU multiply milligrams by 1,660
        For milligrams multiply IU by 0.0006

THE COLORS OF VITAMIN A

Carotenes color autumn leaves, fruits and vegetables. Let color be your guide when choosing fruits and vegetables with the highest vitamin A value. Brightly colored orange, red, yellow and green have the most. Bold green chlorophyll covers up the carotenes, the same way summer green leaves hide the oranges and golds of fall.

You will see the terms carotene and carotenoid used interchangeably to refer to these pigments. Many of the compounds that give color to fruits and vegetables may not have nutritional value as a vitamin but may act as antioxidants.

Beta-carotene is often used as an additive to color foods yellow. About 4 milligrams of beta-carotene is added to a pound of margarine, coloring it yellow to resemble butter and adding to its antioxidant content.

VITAMIN A AND CHILDREN

Vitamin A deficiency is an important health problem in underdeveloped areas of the world. Severe vitamin A deficiency is a major cause of blindness, affecting 500,000 children a year. Less severe deficiencies cause increased incidence of diarrhea and respiratory disease and contribute to increased death from infectious diseases like measles. Supplements of vitamin A dramatically lower the death rate in these children.

The World Health Organization estimates that improved vitamin A intake could prevent between 1.3 million and 2.5 million children's deaths a year.

A CLOSER LOOK AT ANTIOXIDANT VITAMIN C

Vitamin C is an important antioxidant and free radical scavenger in the body. Unlike vitamin E and beta-carotene, which are fat soluble and act in fat tissue, vitamin C is water soluble and found in body fluids. "C" has many important jobs. It is the first line of defense against LDL (low density lipoprotein or "bad" cholesterol) oxidation. Vitamin C also recycles vitamin E, which becomes inactive after acting as an antioxidant. Vitamin C helps maintain levels of vitamin E in the body.

A study, at the University of California at Berkeley, showed that men who ate less vitamin C had a greater chance of fathering children with birth defects and certain types of cancer. The researchers strongly believe vitamin C may protect DNA, the body's blueprint for hereditary traits, from free radical damage, which may result in infertility and damaged sperm. There are serious problems when the DNA blueprint is altered and damage in sperm cells is less likely when vitamin C intake is high.

Older people participating in The Baltimore Longitudinal Study on Aging who had higher body levels of vitamin C also had higher levels of HDL (good) cholesterol. In this way, vitamin C may help protect against heart disease. When HDL is high, the risk for heart attack is low.

Studies show a reduced risk of cancer of the GI tract (gastrointestinal tract) in populations with a high intake of vitamin C. Because vitamin C rich foods also contain other antioxidants, nutrients and fiber, it is hard to be sure if the reduction in cancer is due to vitamin C alone or to all these nutrients working as a team.

When the skin is exposed to the sunlight's ultraviolet irradiation, vitamin C levels in the skin are severely depleted. Using a vitamin C–rich cream protects the skin from free radical damage.

Unhealthy gums are a major cause of tooth loss. Vitamin C keeps gums healthy. In one study, a dose of 600 mg of C reduced gum disease.

Studies show that people who consume the most vitamin C have the lowest blood pressure. The more vitamin C eaten the lower the blood pressure.

Taking vitamin C may make you feel more comfortable when you catch a cold. It acts like an antihistamine to reduce symptoms, such as a stuffy nose, that make a cold sufferer feel miserable.

Vitamin C acts as an antioxidant in food the same way it acts in the body. Manufacturers add C to foods like cured meats, wine, beer, margarine, ice cream and canned fruits and vegetables to protect them from oxygen, which causes discoloration or spoiling. You do the same thing at home when you dip sliced apples into lemon juice to keep them from browning.

How much vitamin C do I need?

Burns, infections, cigarette smoking, aspirin, oral contraceptives and some medications all increase the need for vitamin C. After surgery, supplements of vitamin C are often given to promote healing. After a major operation, as much as 1,000 mg of the vitamin may be needed.

The average vitamin C intake in the United States is 109 milligrams in men and 77 milligrams in women. The Daily Value for vitamin C is 60 mg a day. Smokers are urged to get more—at least 100 mg a day.

Because of the newly appreciated role of vitamin C as an antioxidant, numerous researchers are recommending 250 to 500 milligrams as a better daily target.

Can you have too much vitamin C?

When people take large amounts of vitamin C—over 1 or 2 grams (1,000) or 2,000 mg) a day for a period of time, the body compensates by utilizing less of it. The result is that their body begins to depend on large doses. Taking more than 2 grams (2,000 mg) a day is risky.

Large amounts of vitamin C can cause problems. Nausea, cramps and diarrhea have been reported when people take more than one or two grams a day. In fact some recommendations about this vitamin suggest that you keep increasing the dose until you get diarrhea. Then you know that you are taking enough!

You may have heard that excess vitamin C can't hurt, because the surplus is just passed out in the urine. It's not so simple. Excess vitamin C in the urine can interfere with test results for diabetes and with anticoagulant medications. In people who have a tendency towards gout or an abnormality in the way their body breaks down vitamin C, kidney stones can result.

MEASURING VITAMIN C

Vitamin C is measured in milligrams (mg). There are 1,000 milligrams in a gram. Recommendations for the vitamin on labels give the vitamin content in milligrams.

A CLOSER LOOK AT ANTIOXIDANT VITAMIN E

Since its discovery in 1922, vitamin E has been recommended to fight heart disease, chest pains, pollution, aging, sexual problems, leg cramps, benign breast lumps (fibrocystic disease), menopausal symptoms like hot flashes and vaginal dryness, and more. *Tocopherol*—from the Greek, meaning "to bring forth offspring"—is the chemical name for vitamin E. As a matter of fact the first established use for vitamin E was helping sterile rats reproduce, giving it a reputation as a sex aid.

There are four different tocopherols, forms of vitamin E, found in food—alpha, beta, delta, and gamma. The most active is alpha-tocopherol. This is the one measured in foods and used on labels.

The Daily Value (the amount needed by someone eating 2000 calories a day) found on nutrition labels (see page xl) for vitamin E is 30 IU alpha-tocopherol, and a deficiency is rare. When it occurs, it is usually due to a medical problem rather than too little vitamin E in the diet. If left untreated vitamin E deficiency will cause loss of muscle coordination and reflexes, or impaired vision and speech. Another serious symptom of severe vitamin E deficiency is the breaking open (hemolysis) of red blood cells. This probably is a result of free radical damage to blood cell membranes. Vitamin E supplements correct this condition.

Lumps in the breast that are painful yet benign may respond to treatment with vitamin E supplements. Leg cramps during walking also have been successfully treated with vitamin E.

Benefits of Vitamin E

Vitamin E is one of the body's main defenders against free radicals. It protects body substances from being attacked or oxidized by being hit or oxidized itself. In this way vitamin E protects body fats, cell membranes, lungs, and blood cells from being damaged by free radicals. It also protects beta-carotene, the plant form of vitamin A, from being attacked by free radicals.

Two pollutants—ozone and nitrogen dioxide—produce free radicals that damage the lung tissue when inhaled. Prolonged exposure to air pollution can lead to chronic lung disease. Studies on animals show that vitamin E can protect against this.

While the cause of Parkinson's disease is unknown, it has been is suggested that oxidant stress could be a major factor leading to the neurological degeneration seen in this disease. A pilot study showed that patients could delay taking medication for more than two and one half years when they were given vitamins E and C. Other patients had a reduction in the anxiety and depression common in Parkinson's disease. Another study shows vitamin E supplements reduced the number of seizures in people with epilepsy, underscoring the vitamin's importance in neurological disorders.

There is now accumulating evidence that even healthy people can increase their immune function by taking antioxidant vitamin supplements. A study in Boston showed that when well-nourished men and women aged 60 plus were given 800 IU of vitamin E for 30 days, their immune function improved and they had fewer infections. The researchers believe that this may be a practical way to delay or reverse the decline of immune function that happens as people age. Preliminary results indicate that lower levels of vitamin E work just as well. In another study older adults improved their immune function and reduced infection by 50 percent when they took a multivitamin supplement with extra vitamin E and C.

Vitamin E reduces the frequency and severity of menopausal hot flashes, enhances energy and provides a sense of well-being. For many the vitamin has even relieved uncomfortable vaginal dryness. Some dermatologists recommend rubbing vitamin E oil on injured skin to prevent scarring. Oncologists often recommend applying vitamin E to relieve mouth sores resulting from chemotherapy. Though popularly accepted, these benefits of vitamin E have not yet been scientifically proven. The evidence, though, is beginning to accumulate.

Vitamin E and the Heart

Scientists think that low-density lipoproteins (LDL), popularly called "bad" cholesterol, are a risk factor for heart attack when they have been oxidized. Oxidation changes them so that they stick to the artery walls, narrowing arteries and interfering with blood flow. A heart attack can follow. Many studies show that large amounts of vitamin E can help prevent the oxidation of LDL.

A study done at the University of Texas Southwestern Medical Center in Dallas showed that the LDL cholesterol of men who were given 800 IU of vitamin E a day was only half as likely to be oxidized as the LDL in those men receiving no supplements. Getting this much vitamin E from foods isn't possible without overloading on fat and calories because the richest sources of vitamin E are vegetable oils, wheat germ, nuts, and seeds.

The good news is that smaller amounts of vitamin E may benefit the heart too. Two recent, large studies, where over 120,000 men and women were followed for four to eight years, showed that vitamin E supplementation reduced the risk of heart disease by 40 percent. This is dramatic proof that vitamin E is good for the heart.

A European study showed that patients with chest pains (angina) had lower blood levels of vitamin E than others who had no chest pain. The relationship between lower vitamin E and chest pain continued even when smoking was taken into account.

In a multinational study sponsored by the World Health Organization, high levels of vitamin E were found in populations with fewer deaths from heart disease. The benefit seen was believed due to the teamwork among vitamins E, C and the plant form of vitamin A. The better the overall antioxidant status for all three of them, the lower the death rate. But most research points to vitamin E as the most protective.

How much vitamin E do I need?

Although frank deficiency of vitamin E is rare and seen only in premature babies or people who do not absorb fat normally, average intakes of vitamin E in the United States, 9.6 milligrams for men and 7 milligrams for women, fall short of the recommended amount. Many experts feel 100 IU of vitamin E are needed daily for maximum antioxidant protection. Many foods rich in vitamin E are also high in fat. Increasing the intake of foods like oils, nuts, eggs, doughnuts and cakes will greatly increase fat intake while providing more vitamin E. Eating more fruits and vegetables not only increases vitamin E but also vitamins C, the plant form of vitamin A and fiber. Unfortunately, it is not easy to get 100 IU of vitamin E in that way. This is one time when supplements may be called for.

Even though vitamin E is found in many foods, the average person can't get enough to supply the amounts shown to be needed as an antioxidant. Highly fortified cereals and instant breakfasts often have vitamin E content equal to 20 milligrams. Even using these products regularly cannot ensure intakes of 100 IU daily. This is the lowest level studies show to be protective against heart disease.

Can you have too much vitamin E?

As much as 3200 IU a day taken for as long as six months has been shown by scientifically controlled studies to have very few adverse side effects. In fact, there was no single negative side effect from vitamin E that showed up in every study. That's important because when side effects are not consistent from one study to another, researchers assume the side effects have nothing to do with the vitamin.

There is one caution that must be considered before you take high doses of vitamin E. It can be a problem for people who are already taking anticoagulant medication because

---

MEASURING VITAMIN E

Vitamin E is available in both natural and synthetic forms. It can be measured in milligrams and International Units (IU). The synthetic form is less potent than the natural, so a greater amount is needed to equal the vitamin activity of the natural form. Vitamin supplements made with synthetic vitamin E contain slightly more vitamin E so as to equal the potency of natural vitamin E.

Vitamin E, natural	1 IU = 1.5 milligrams
Vitamin E, synthetic	1 IU = 1 milligram

high doses of vitamin E may make the blood take longer to clot. If a person is deficient in vitamin K, which is needed for normal blood clotting, adding too much E on top of this problem could make the blood take so long to clot that it would be unsafe. Vitamin E does not cause clotting problems in people who are not taking anticoagulants and are not vitamin K deficient.

ANTIOXIDANT TEAMWORK

Antioxidants often work as a team, protecting different parts of the body. Inside the cells, they protect internal structures; outside the cells, they circulate through the body, mopping up free radicals.

Researchers are beginning to believe that antioxidant teamwork may be more important than the function of the

---

ANTIOXIDANTS AND ATHLETICS

Regular exercise increases the body's production of antioxidants, but at the same time exercise causes muscle damage and increased levels of free radicals. This reduces vitamin E levels in the muscles.

Giving vitamin E and C supplements to endurance athletes reduces tissue damage and speeds up the recovery of muscles from any damage that has occurred. In a recent study, researchers at Washington University School of Medicine gave young male athletes supplements of vitamins E, C and beta-carotene. Those taking the supplements formed 17% to 36% fewer free radicals than other athletes who took a placebo.

"Weekend Warriors" may be at even greater risk. Sporadic bouts of athletics put their bodies under severe oxidative stress. They may need even more antioxidants than a person who exercises regularly.

individual players. Some studies that show benefits from beta-carotene and vitamin E individually show added benefits when there are high body levels of vitamin C as well. Recent research showed that combining vitamins E, C and the plant form of vitamin A resulted in increased body levels of these antioxidants and reduced the risk of heart disease. A study comparing people with and without cataracts showed that those who took more supplements of vitamins C and E had fewer cataracts.

It may be that each antioxidant acts differently, offering protection in a different way. By acting together, these benefits are magnified. The value of this teamwork may be greater than what we know now. A more complete understanding

---

IMMUNE-FRIENDLY NUTRIENTS

Your immune system protects your body against invading viruses, bacteria, parasites or fungi. These microorganisms are first thwarted by physical obstacles like the skin. If this line of defense is crossed, another system is activated. An army of cells in the blood masses to fight the invaders.

The antioxidant nutrients support these cells in their battle against the microscopic invaders. Many researchers believe that eating more antioxidant-rich foods will enhance this immune response.

VITAMIN A, PLANT SOURCES: carrots, sweet potatoes, cantaloupe, apricots, spinach, broccoli, winter squash

VITAMIN C: oranges, broccoli, sweet potatoes, red and green peppers, turnip greens, Brussels sprouts, cauliflower, kiwi, strawberries, cantaloupe

VITAMIN E: wheat germ, vegetable oil, brown rice, almonds, whole wheat, oats, yeast

may take many years, but it really isn't necessary to completely understand how antioxidants work to benefit from them. What is clear at this point is that eating more antioxidant foods, those rich in vitamins A, C, and E, can help protect health. There is no risk, only benefit, in choosing healthy, antioxidant-rich foods.

SMOKING AND ANTIOXIDANTS

Smokers have lower levels of antioxidants—vitamins C, E and the plant form of vitamin A in their bodies. Cigarette smoke contains toxic compounds that can increase the damage done by free radicals. Smoking also inactivates vitamin E reducing its ability to protect the lungs. This may be a major contributor to lung disease and lung cancer.

Even nonsmokers are at risk. Passive women smokers—those who are exposed to other people's cigarette smoke for at least 20 hours a week—have lower levels of vitamin C similar to women smokers. It may be worthwhile for passive smokers to increase their vitamin C intake and follow the same advice given to women who smoke.

Even when smokers eat the same amount of fruits and vegetables as nonsmokers they have lower amounts of the plant form of vitamin A in their blood. Eating more fruits and vegetables does not significantly change this.

Did you know . . . ?

The ancient Egyptians preserved dead bodies by embalming them with oils and plant extracts that acted as antioxidants.

The basic chemicals of life may have been formed by free radical reactions that were fueled by radiation from the sun. Scientists theorize that life arose spontaneously as a result.

INCREASING ANTIOXIDANTS

IN THE SUPERMARKET

Next time you shop at the supermarket, think antioxidants! Begin with produce to boost your antioxidant total. Round out these choices with frozen and canned fruits and vegetables. Don't forget dried fruits, seeds and nuts. Dress your salad with a vitamin E–rich oil and toss in some chickpeas or soybeans. Stock up on wheat germ, whole grain breads and cereals. Take home a large supply of vitamin C–rich juices and beverages.

Become a label reader. Nutrition labels, which are becoming more widely used due to the federal Nutrition Labeling and Education Act, can help you make the best antioxidant choices. This new legislation, which becomes effective in May 1994, will require every food package bigger than a Lifesaver roll to carry a "Nutrition Facts" panel. The new nutrition panel on food labels will be called "Nutrition Facts," replacing the old label called "Nutrition Information." Look for the new name to signal that the label you are reading meets the new NLEA regulations.

The whole purpose of the law is to make the nutrition label more useful for consumers and allow them to compare between similar brands. Listings for the antioxidant vitamins A and C are mandatory, but it is up to the manufacturer to decide whether or not to list vitamin E since this is voluntary.

All vitamins and minerals will be listed as a percentage of the **Daily Value.** Daily Value, or DV, is the amount of that vitamin or mineral needed by someone eating 2000 calories a day. Though this guidepost is not for everyone, it does allow you to find out if a food is rich or poor in a vitamin or mineral. The higher the Daily Value percentage the richer a food is in that vitamin or mineral. The legal definition of an "excellent" or "rich" source is a food that contains 20% or more of the Daily Value in one serving. A "good" source has at least 10%.

Antioxidants	Per Serving Rich Source	Good Source
Vitamin A (plant source)	1000 IU or more	500 IU
Vitamin C	12 mg or more	6 mg
Vitamin E	6 IU or more	3 IU

ADD FLAVOR, ADD ANTIOXIDANTS

Seasonings like garlic, nutmeg, cloves, rosemary, ginger, oregano, pepper and thyme are natural antioxidants and act as natural preservatives.

Garlic is a potent antioxidant. Studies show it reduces the oxidation of LDL (low density lipoproteins), an early risk factor for heart disease. It also reduces the fats in blood, triglycerides and cholesterol that are linked to heart disease. Seven to 28 cloves of garlic a day lowers cholesterol and decreases blood clotting, reducing risk of heart attack and stroke. In Germany, a garlic preparation is a licensed drug for atherosclerosis, a major risk factor for heart disease. Garlic also lowers blood pressure and blood sugar.

Many studies have shown antioxidants in food protect against cancer. Studies in China and Italy found that when diets are rich in garlic, stomach cancer is reduced. In studies on animals, garlic reduces lung cancer.

Miso, Japanese soybean paste, is an antioxidant. When soy is fermented to make soy sauce, a compound is produced that reduces esophageal cancer in mice.

Peppermint, spearmint and other members of the mint family are rich sources of antioxidants.

Nutrition labeling will not only appear on package labels, the law is also recommending voluntary point-of-purchase nutrition labeling for the 20 most commonly eaten fruits and vegetables. Because fruits and vegetables are rich in antioxidants, this information will be very helpful. The following two charts list the 20 most commonly eaten fruits and the 20 most commonly eaten vegetables, showing if each is an "excellent," "good" or "minor source" of antioxidants.

20 MOST COMMONLY EATEN FRUITS

(R = Rich source; G = Good source; M = Minor source)

Food	Vitamin A			Vitamin C			Vitamin E		
	R	G	M	R	G	M	R	G	M
Banana			X			X			X
Apple			X			X			X
Watermelon (⅛)	X					X			X
Orange (Navel, Valencia, Florida)			X			X			X
Cantaloupe (½)	X					X			X
Grapes (20)			X			X			X
Grapefruit (½) Pink, Red, White			X			X			X
Strawberries (1 cup)			X			X			X
Peach		X				X			X
Pear			X			X			X
Nectarine	X					X			X
Honeydew (⅒)			X		X				X
Plum			X		X				X
Avocado (½)		X				X			X
Lemon			X	X					X
Pineapple (½ cup)			X	X					X
Tangerine	X					X			X
Cherries (20)			X		X				X
Kiwifruit			X	X					X
Lime			X	X					X

20 MOST COMMONLY EATEN VEGETABLES

(R = Rich source; G = Good source; M = Minor source)

Vegetable	Vitamin A R	Vitamin A G	Vitamin A M	Vitamin C R	Vitamin C G	Vitamin C M	Vitamin E R	Vitamin E G	Vitamin E M
Potato			X	X					X
Iceberg Lettuce			X			X			X
(5 leaves)									
Tomato		X		X					X
Onion			X		X				X
Carrot	X			X					X
Celery (1 stalk)			X			X			X
Sweet Corn (1 ear)			X			X			X
Broccoli (½ cup)		X		X					X
Green Cabbage (½ cup)			X	X					X
Cucumber									
(1 large)			X	X					X
(½ cup sliced)			X			X			X
Bell Pepper									
Green			X	X					X
Red	X			X					X
Cauliflower (½ cup)			X	X					X
Leaf Lettuce (½ cup shredded)		X				X			X
Sweet Potato	X			X					X
Mushroom									
(1 whole)			X			X			X
(½ cup sliced)			X			X			X
Scallions									
(1 tablespoon)			X			X			X
(½ cup)			X			X			X
Green (Snap) Beans (½ cup)			X		X				X
Radishes (10)			X		X				X
Summer Squash (½ cup)									
Crookneck			X			X			X
Zucchini			X		X				X
Asparagus (½ cup)			X		X				X

What is obvious from the preceding tables is that although fruits and vegetables can be good to rich sources of the antioxidant vitamins A and C, none are excellent sources of vitamin E. Oils, nuts and wheat germ are the richest sources of this important antioxidant. It is not wise for anyone to increase their intake of oils simply to get more vitamin E but both wheat germ and small servings of nuts can provide tasty antioxidant-rich additions to your meals.

VITAMIN E FOUND IN NUTS AND WHEAT GERM

	Vitamin E (IU)
Nuts (1 ounce)	
Brazil nuts	2
Almonds	
dried	6
honey roasted	6
oil roasted	2
toasted	14
Filberts	7
Peanuts	2
Pecans	1
Walnuts	1
Wheat Germ (¼ cup)	6

IN THE KITCHEN

Some of the antioxidant vitamins are lost during cooking. That's why raw fruits and vegetables are good choices. But when you cook, you can prevent their total loss by

- Reducing the water used for cooking.
- Reducing the cooking time—keep it short.
- Leaving the food in large pieces.

Steaming and microwaving are better than boiling. Cooked crisp is better than overcooking. Cooking the whole fruit or vegetable is better than cutting it up. The smaller the pieces the greater the vitamin loss.

If you bake a whole potato in its skin you lose only 20% of its vitamin C. Boiled without the skin, almost 50% is lost. Peel, boil and mash the potato and 75% of the vitamin C is destroyed.

Heating oils reduces their vitamin E content, destroying as much as 99 percent of its vitamin E.

Soaking is another way to lose vitamins. Don't soak vegetables or salad greens. Keeping fruits and vegetables chilled preserves antioxidants. The fruit bowl on the kitchen counter may be pretty but keeping fruit in the refrigerator crisper saves the vitamins. Vitamin C–rich juice should be stored refrigerated, in a covered opaque container. Don't leave it on the breakfast table—pour and store.

Frozen foods should be kept solidly frozen and used within a month or two. Even canned foods can lose vitamins during storage. Don't bury them in the back of the cupboard. Vitamin losses double in canned foods when temperatures reach 80°F or above. Don't store canned foods next to the stove and use foods more quickly during the summer. To preserve antioxidants, prepare foods as close to the time they will be eaten as possible.

Cooking in glass, stainless steel, aluminum, enamel or plastic preserves antioxidant vitamins. Copper destroys vitamins C and E. Copper cooking pots should be lined with another metal. Iron pots destroy vitamin C.

HOW GREEN IS YOUR SALAD?

Green vegetables, especially the leafy kind, are rich in the antioxidant vitamins A and C. Having a large **green** salad daily is a delicious way to add antioxidants to your diet. Look for seasonal varieties or try some of the more unusual choices next time you shop. (See the table on the facing page.)

Tips for Enriching Your Recipes with Antioxidants:

- Use a vitamin E–rich oil in place of solid fat.
- Use a vitamin E–rich oil to make salad dressing.
- Substitute fruit puree for ½ the fat or oil in baked products. (Buy baby food prunes, mangos, apricots, peaches or drain and puree canned varieties.)
- Add wheat germ to baked products, casseroles, meatballs, soups and pancakes.
- Use ½ cup wheat germ to replace ½ cup flour in muffins. (Add 2 tablespoons of water to keep them moist.)
- Use ¼ cup wheat germ to replace ¼ cup flour in a single pie crust.
- Use 1 cup wheat germ to replace 1 cup flour in cookies.
- Use almonds when nuts are called for.
- Substitute orange juice or another vitamin C–rich juice when fruit juice is used.
- Substitute chopped prunes, peaches or apricots when raisins are called for.
- Use warmed fruit purees instead of gravy.
- Substitute whole wheat flour for ½ the flour in recipes.

ADD A DASH OF ANTIOXIDANT

A number of common herbs are rich in carotenoids, the plant form of vitamin A. Adding some to a favorite recipe is another way to make your diet antioxidant rich.

HERB	PORTION	VIT A (IU)
basil, dry	1 tsp	131
chives, fresh	1 tbsp	137
cilantro	¼ cup	111
parsley, dry	1 tbsp	252
fresh	1 tbsp	520

	VIT C (MG)	VIT A (IU)
arugula (rocket), chopped, ½ cup	237	—
avocado, ¼	308	4
bok choy, shredded, ½ cup	1050	16
borage, chopped, ½ cup	1848	15
broccoli, ½ cup	678	41
cabbage, raw shredded, ½ cup		
pak-choi	1050	16
pe-tsai	912	21
savoy	350	11
chicory, chopped, ½ cup	3600	22
chives, chopped, 2 tablespoons	262	4
collards, chopped, ½ cup	599	4
dandelion greens, chopped, ½ cup	3920	10
dock, chopped, ½ cup	2680	32
endive, chopped, ½ cup	513	2
garden cress, chopped, ½ cup	2325	17
green onions (scallions), sliced, ¼ cup	97	5
green pepper, sliced, ½ cup	316	45
kale, chopped, ½ cup	3026	41
lettuce		
Boston, 6 leaves	876	6
iceberg, 6 leaves	396	6
looseleaf, shredded, ½ cup	532	5
romaine, shredded, ½ cup	728	7
mustard greens, chopped, ½ cup	1484	20
parsley, chopped, ¼ cup	780	20
pokeberry shoots, chopped, ½ cup	6960	109
purslane, chopped, ½ cup	284	5
spinach, chopped, ½ cup	1880	8
swamp cabbage, chopped, ½ cup	1764	16
Swiss chard, chopped, ½ cup	594	5
watercress, chopped, ½ cup	799	7
zucchini, sliced, ½ cup	221	6

all values given are for raw, fresh vegetables
— means no values available

Try these antioxidant-rich muffins. Ingredients in bold type are good antioxidant sources.

ANTI-O MUFFINS

1 cup flour	1 tbsp baking powder
½ cup **whole wheat flour**	½ tsp baking soda
½ cup **wheat germ**	1 cup **orange juice**
⅓ cup brown sugar	⅓ cup **apricot or mango puree***
½ cup chopped **dried apricots**	1 egg
¼ cup chopped **almonds**	1 tsp vanilla
1 tbsp grated lemon rind	

Preheat oven to 425° F.

Spray muffin pans with cooking spray.

In a large bowl combine flour, whole wheat flour, wheat germ, brown sugar, peaches, almonds, lemon rind, baking powder and baking soda.

In a two-cup measure combine orange juice, apricot puree, egg and vanilla.

Pour liquid ingredients into flour mixture, stirring only to combine; mixture will be lumpy. Spoon into muffin pans; bake at 425°F for 20 to 25 minutes. Remove from pan to cool. Makes 12 muffins.

* Buy strained baby fruits or drain and puree canned. Nutrition Analysis Per Muffin: 150 Calories, 15% Fat, 2490 IU Vitamin A, 11 mg Vitamin C, 3 IU Vitamin E

Now it's your turn to count your antioxidants. Note everything you eat today, then look up each food you have eaten in Parts I and II to see how much vitamin A and vitamin C is in the food and then look it up in Part III and see how much vitamin E you ate today. Because many foods have not been analyzed for vitamin E, you may not be able to find the food you have eaten. This isn't a problem because it is very difficult, if not impossible, for most of us to get our target intake of vitamin E from food alone. An exception to

A SAMPLE DAY OF ANTIOXIDANT-RICH FOOD CHOICES

	VITAMINS		
	A (IU plant source)	C (mg)	E (IU)
BREAKFAST			
Orange juice (1 cup)	194	97	—
Oatmeal, instant (1 pkg)	1237	0	tr
Wheat Germ (2 tbsp)	17	0	5
Lowfat Milk (½ cup)	250	1	—
Anti-o Muffin	2490	11	3
Coffee	—	—	—
LUNCH			
Chicken Broth (1 bowl)	tr	tr	tr
Egg Salad (½ cup)	578	—	12
Lettuce (2 leaves)	132	2	tr
Corn Stick (2)	104	tr	tr
Mineral water	—	—	—
SNACK			
Graham Honey Cookies (3)	tr	2	3
Apricots, dried (5 halves)	1267	15	—
Lemonade (1 cup)	53	10	—
DINNER			
Cantaloupe (½)	8608	113	—
Chicken Cacciatore (¾ cup)	1586	40	8
Pasta (2 ounces)	0	0	4
Asparagus (4 spears)	491	15	1
Chocolate Pudding (4 oz)	182	1	3
Tea	0	0	—
SNACK			
Orange Sherbet (½ cup)	93	2	—
TOTAL	17282	309	39

— indicates no value is available

VITAMIN	SUGGESTED DAILY INTAKE	INTAKE FROM FOOD
A	5000 IU	4000 IU from plant sources
C	250–500 MG	250 MG
E	100–200 IU	15–25 IU

this might be if you eat large amounts of highly fortified cereal daily. Some of these cereals contain 30 IU in a cup. Two cups added to the foods listed in the sample day would just meet the suggested daily intake for vitamin E.

USING YOUR ANTIOXIDANT COUNTER

The Antioxidant Vitamin Counter is divided into three main sections. Parts I and II list the vitamin A and C values in generic, brand name, take-out and fast foods. Part III lists vitamin E values because a more limited number of values are available for vitamin E. Over 7,000 foods are represented in these two lists. For example, when you want to select an oil, look up the oil category on page 252. You will find nineteen different oils listed so you can see which one is the best source of vitamin E.

Foods are listed alphabetically. For each group, you will find brand name foods listed first in alphabetical order, followed by an alphabetical listing of generic foods. Large categories are divided into subcategories—canned, fresh, frozen, and ready-to-use to make it easier to find what you are looking for.

Most foods are listed alphabetically. But, in some cases, foods are grouped by category. For example, pasta dinners, like spaghetti and meatballs, lasagna and manicotti are all found under the category PASTA DISHES. Other group categories include:

DINNERS   Page 72
    Includes all frozen dinners by brand
    name

ICE CREAM AND FROZEN DESSERTS   Page 97
    Includes all dairy and non-dairy ice
    cream and frozen novelties

ANTIOXIDANT COUNTING
A SAMPLE WORKSHEET

BREAKFAST	A (IU Plant source)	Vitamins C mg	E IU

Breakfast

Snack

Lunch

Snack

Dinner

Snack

	Total	_____	_____	_____

VITAMIN	SUGGESTED DAILY INTAKE	INTAKE FROM FOOD
A	5000 IU	4000 IU from plant sources
C	250–500 MG	250 MG
E	100–200 IU	15–25 IU

Iii INTRODUCTION

DEFINITIONS

as prep (as prepared): refers to food that has been prepared according to package directions

cooked: refers to food cooked without the addition of fat (oil, butter, margarine, etc.); steaming, poaching, broiling and dry roasting are examples of this type of preparation

generic: describes a food without a brand name

home recipe: describes homemade dishes; those included can be used as guide to the cholesterol and calorie values of similar products you may prepare or take-out food you buy ready-to-eat

lean and fat: describes meat with some fat on its edges that is not cut away before cooking or poultry prepared with skin and fat as purchased

lean only: lean portion, trimmed of all visible fat

shelf stable or **shelf ready:** refers to prepared products found on the supermarket shelf that are ready to be heated and do not require refrigeration

take-out: describes prepared dishes that you purchase ready-to-eat; those included serve as a guide to the vitamin and calorie values of similar products you may purchase

trace (tr): value use when a food contains less than one calorie or less than one mg of vitamin C or less than 1 IU of vitamins A or E

ABBREVIATIONS

avg	=	average
diam	=	diameter
frzn	=	frozen
g	=	gram
lb	=	pound
lg	=	large
med	=	medium
mg	=	milligram
oz	=	ounce
pkg	=	package
pt	=	pint
prep	=	prepared
reg	=	regular
sm	=	small
sq	=	square
tbsp	=	tablespoon
tr	=	trace
tsp	=	teaspoon
w/	=	with
w/o	=	without
in	=	inch
<	=	less than

EQUIVALENT MEASURES

1 tablespoon	=	3 teaspoons
4 tablespoons	=	¼ cup
8 tablespoons	=	½ cup
12 tablespoons	=	¾ cup
16 tablespoons	=	1 cup
1000 milligrams	=	1 gram
28 grams	=	1 ounce

Liquid Measurements

2 tablespoons	=	1 ounce
¼ cup	=	2 ounces
½ cup	=	4 ounces
¾ cup	=	6 ounces
1 cup	=	8 ounces
2 cups	=	1 pint
4 cups	=	1 quart

Dry Measurements

16 ounces	=	1 pound
12 ounces	=	¾ pound
8 ounces	=	½ pound
4 ounces	=	¼ pound

Discrepancies in figures are due to rounding, product reformulation and reevaluation.

PART I

Vitamin A and Vitamin C Values for Brand-Name and Generic Foods

ALL VITAMIN A VALUES ARE GIVEN IN INTERNATIONAL UNITS (IU).
ALL VITAMIN C VALUES ARE GIVEN IN MILLIGRAMS (MG).

FOOD	PORTION	CAL	VIT A	VIT C

ACEROLA

FRESH
| acerola | 1 | 2 | 37 | 81 |

JUICE
| juice | 1 cup | 51 | 1232 | 3872 |

ADZUKI BEANS

DRIED
| cooked | 1 cup | 294 | 13 | 0 |

AKEE

| fresh | 3.5 oz | 223 | 1 | 26 |

ALFALFA

| sprouts | 1 cup | 40 | 51 | 3 |
| sprouts | 1 tbsp | 1 | 5 | tr |

ALLSPICE

| ground | 1 tsp | 5 | 10 | 1 |

ALMONDS

almond butter w/ honey & cinnamon	1 tbsp	96	0	tr
almond butter w/ salt	1 tbsp	101	0	tr
almond butter w/o salt	1 tbsp	101	0	tr
almond paste	1 oz	127	0	tr
dried, blanched	1 oz	166	0	tr
dried, unblanched	1 oz	167	0	tr
dry roasted, unblanched	1 oz	167	0	tr
dry roasted, unblanched, salted	1 oz	167	0	tr
oil roasted, blanched	1 oz	174	0	tr
oil roasted, blanched, salted	1 oz	174	0	tr

FOOD	PORTION	CAL	VIT A	VIT C
oil roasted, unblanched	1 oz	176	0	tr
toasted, unblanched	1 oz	167	0	tr

AMARANTH

FOOD	PORTION	CAL	VIT A	VIT C
Amaranth Cereal With Bananas (Health Valley)	½ cup (1 oz)	110	160	1
Amaranth Crunch With Raisins (Health Valley)	¼ cup (1 oz)	110	7	tr
Amaranth Flakes 100% Organic (Health Valley)	½ cup (1 oz)	90	26	1
Fast Menu Amaranth With Garden Vegetables (Health Valley)	7.5 oz	140	5010	5
cooked	½ cup	59	1828	27

APPLE

FOOD	PORTION	CAL	VIT A	VIT C
CANNED				
applesauce, sweetened	½ cup	97	14	2
applesauce, unsweetened	½ cup	53	35	2
sliced, sweetened	1 cup	136	103	1
DRIED				
cooked w/ sugar	½ cup	116	22	1
cooked w/o sugar	½ cup	172	22	1
rings	10	155	0	3
FRESH				
apple	1	81	74	8
w/o skin, sliced	1 cup	62	48	4
w/o skin, sliced & cooked	1 cup	91	75	tr
w/o skin, sliced & microwaved	1 cup	96	68	tr
FROZEN				
sliced w/o sugar	½ cup	41	29	tr
JUICE				
Bruce Lite	½ cup	88	6000	9
apple	1 cup	116	2	2

FOOD	PORTION	CAL	VIT A	VIT C
APRICOTS				
CANNED				
Halves Unsweetened (S&W)	½ cup	35	700	2
Halves Diet (S&W)	½ cup	35	750	12
Halves Unpeeled In Heavy Syrup (S&W)	½ cup	110	1750	2
Whole Peeled Diet (S&W)	½ cup	28	750	12
Whole Peeled In Heavy Syrup (S&W)	½ cup	100	1750	2
halves, heavy syrup pack w/ skin	1 cup (9.1 oz)	214	3174	8
halves, water pack w/ skin	1 cup (8.5 oz)	65	3142	8
halves, water pack w/o skin	1 cup (8 oz)	51	4109	4
heavy syrup w/ skin	3 halves	70	1046	3
juice pack w/ skin	3 halves	40	1421	4
light syrup w/ skin	3 halves	54	1124	2
puree juice pack w/ skin	1 cup (8.7 oz)	119	4195	12
puree from heavy syrup pack w/ skin	¾ cup (9.1 oz)	214	3174	8
puree from light pack w/ skin	¾ cup (8.9 oz)	160	3344	7
puree from water pack w/ skin	¾ cup (8.5 oz)	65	3142	8
water pack w/ skin	3 halves	22	1086	3
water pack w/o skin	4 halves	20	1629	2
DRIED				
halves	10	83	2534	1
halves, cooked w/o sugar	½ cup	106	2954	2
FRESH				
apricots	3	51	2769	11
FROZEN				
sweetened	½ cup	119	2033	11
JUICE				
Kern's Nectar	6 oz	100	2200	27

FOOD	PORTION	CAL	VIT A	VIT C
S&W Nectar	6 oz	35	2000	1
nectar	1 cup	141	3304	1

ARROWROOT

flour	1 cup	457	0	0

ARTICHOKE

CANNED

FOOD	PORTION	CAL	VIT A	VIT C
Hearts Marinated (S&W)	½ cup	225	100	10
FRESH Dole	1 lg	23	0	7
boiled	1 med (4 oz)	60	212	12
hearts, cooked	½ cup	42	149	8
jerusalem, raw, sliced	½ cup	57	15	3
FROZEN Hearts Deluxe (Birds Eye)	½ cup	30	100	5
cooked	1 pkg (9 oz)	108	394	12

ASPARAGUS

CANNED

FOOD	PORTION	CAL	VIT A	VIT C
Points Water Pack (S&W)	½ cup	17	500	21
Spears Colossal Fancy (S&W)	½ cup	20	500	15
Spears Fancy (S&W)	½ cup	18	500	15
FRESH Dole	5 spears	18	604	9
cooked	½ cup	22	485	18
cooked	4 spears	14	323	7
raw	½ cup	16	390	9
raw	4 spears	14	338	8
FROZEN Big Valley	2.7 oz	23	800	26
Cut (Birds Eye)	½ cup	23	1000	27

FOOD	PORTION	CAL	VIT A	VIT C
Harvest Fresh Cuts (Green Giant)	½ cup	25	500	12
Spears (Birds Eye)	½ cup	25	750	30
cooked	1 pkg (10 oz)	82	2397	72
cooked	4 spears	17	491	15

AVOCADO
FRESH
avocado	1	324	1230	16
puree	1 cup	370	1407	18

BACON
cooked	3 strips	109	0	6
gammon, lean & fat, grilled	4.2 oz	274	0	0
grilled	2 slices (1.7 oz)	86	0	10

BACON SUBSTITUTE
bacon substitute	1 strip	25	7	0

BAGEL
FRESH
cinnamon raisin	1 (3.5 in)	194	52	1
cinnamon raisin, toasted	1 (3.5 in)	194	47	tr
egg	1 (3.5 in)	197	77	tr
egg, toasted	1 (3.5 in)	197	70	tr
oat bran	1 (3.5 in)	181	3	tr
oat bran, toasted	1 (3.5 in)	181	3	tr
onion	1 (3.5 in)	195	0	0
plain	1 (3.5 in)	195	0	0
plain, toasted	1 (3.5 in)	195	0	0
poppy seed	1 (3.5 in)	195	0	0

FOOD	PORTION	CAL	VIT A	VIT C
FROZEN				
Ham & Cheese On A Bagel (Great Starts)	3 oz	240	300	4

BAKING POWDER

baking powder	1 tsp	2	0	0
low sodium	1 tsp	5	0	0

BAKING SODA

baking soda	1 tsp	0	0	0

BALSAM PEAR

leafy tips, cooked	½ cup	10	503	16
leafy tips, raw	½ cup	7	416	21
pods, cooked	½ cup	12	70	21

BAMBOO SHOOTS

CANNED				
sliced	1 cup	25	11	1
FRESH				
cooked	½ cup	15	0	0
raw	½ cup	21	15	3

BANANA

DRIED				
powder	1 tbsp	21	19	tr
FRESH				
Dole	1	120	70	11
banana	1	105	92	10
mashed	1 cup	207	182	20

BARLEY

Quaker Medium Pearled	¼ cup	172	11	0
Quaker Quick Pearled	¼ cup	172	11	0

FOOD	PORTION	CAL	VIT A	VIT C
Scotch Medium Pearled	¼ cup	172	11	0
Scotch Quick Pearled	¼ cup	172	11	0
pearled, uncooked	½ cup	352	22	0

BASIL
ground	1 tsp	4	131	1

BAY LEAF
crumbled	1 tsp	2	37	tr

BEANS
(Some of the bean products contain meat, which contributes a small amount of non-plant vitamin A.)

CANNED				
Baked Beans (Van Camp's)	1 cup	260	0	0
Barbecue Beans (Campbell)	½ can (7⅞ oz)	210	500	5
Barbecue Beans Texas Style (S&W)	½ cup	135	400	2
Big John's Beans 'n Fixin's (Hunt's)	4 oz	170	40	9
Boston Baked (Health Valley)	7.5 oz	190	304	15
Boston Baked No Salt Added (Health Valley)	7.5 oz	190	304	15
Brown Sugar Beans (Van Camp's)	1 cup	290	0	0
Chili (Gebhardt)	4 oz	115	3	4
Deluxe Baked Beans (Van Camp's)	1 cup	320	0	0
Fast Menu Honey Baked Organic Beans With Tofu Weiner (Health Valley)	7.5 oz	150	5000	0
Home Style Beans (Campbell)	½ can (8 oz)	220	300	5
Hot Chili Beans (Campbell)	½ can (7.75 oz)	180	750	6
Mexican Style Chili Beans (Van Camp's)	1 cup	210	1595	1

FOOD	PORTION	CAL	VIT A	VIT C
Mixed Bean Salad Marinated (S&W)	½ cup	90	200	2
Old Fashioned Beans In Molasses & Brown Sugar Sauce (Campbell)	½ can (8 oz)	230	100	6
Pork & Beans In Tomato Sauce (Campbell)	½ can (8 oz)	200	500	2
Pork 'N Beans (S&W)	½ cup	130	100	2
Pork And Beans (Hunt's)	4 oz	135	20	2
Pork and Beans (Van Camp's)	1 cup	216	164	2
Pork and Beans In Tomato Sauce (Green Giant)	½ cup	90	0	0
Refried (Casa Fiesta)	3.5 oz	110	131	6
Refried Jalapeno (Gebhardt)	4 oz	115	8	2
Smokey Ranch Beans (S&W)	½ cup	130	750	2
Three Bean Salad (Green Giant)	½ cup	70	100	0
Vegetarian Means With Miso (Health Valley)	7.5 oz	180	2555	tr
Vegetarian Style (Van Camp's)	1 cup	206	179	2
baked beans w/ beef	½ cup	161	283	2
baked beans w/ franks	½ cup	182	197	3
baked beans w/ pork	½ cup	133	255	3
baked beans w/ pork & sweet sauce	½ cup	140	144	4
baked beans w/ pork & tomato sauce	½ cup	123	156	4
TAKE-OUT				
baked beans	½ cup	190	0	1
barbecue beans	3.5 oz	120	200	2
four-bean salad	3.5 oz	100	500	5
refried beans	½ cup	43	231	0
three-bean salad	¾ cup	230	220	3

FOOD	PORTION	CAL	VIT A	VIT C
BEEF				
FRESH				
bottom round, lean & fat, trim 0 in, Choice, roasted	3 oz	172	0	0
bottom round, lean & fat, trim 0 in, Select, braised	3 oz	171	0	0
bottom round, lean & fat, trim 0 in, Select, roasted	3 oz	150	0	0
bottom round, lean & fat, trim 0 in, braised	3 oz	193	0	0
bottom round, lean & fat, trim ¼ in, Choice, braised	3 oz	241	0	0
bottom round, lean & fat, trim ¼ in, Choice, roasted	3 oz	221	0	0
bottom round, lean & fat, trim ¼ in, Select, braised	3 oz	220	0	0
bottom round, lean & fat, trim ¼ in, Select, roasted	3 oz	199	0	0
brisket flat, half lean & fat, trim 0 in, braised	3 oz	183	0	0
brisket flat, half lean & fat, trim ¼ in, braised	3 oz	309	0	0
brisket point, half lean & fat, trim 0 in, braised	3 oz	304	0	0
brisket point, half lean & fat, trim ¼ in, braised	3 oz	343	0	0
brisket whole, lean & fat, trim 0 in, braised	3 oz	247	0	0
brisket whole, lean & fat, trim ¼ in, braised	3 oz	327	0	0
chuck arm pot roast, lean & fat, trim 0 in, braised	3 oz	238	0	0
chuck arm pot roast, lean & fat, trim ¼ in, braised	3 oz	282	0	0
chuck blade roast, lean & fat, trim 0 in, braised	3 oz	284	0	0

FOOD	PORTION	CAL	VIT A	VIT C
chuck blade roast, lean & fat, trim ¼ in, braised	3 oz	293	0	0
eye of round, lean & fat, trim 0 in, Choice, roasted	3 oz	153	0	0
eye of round, lean & fat, trim 0 in, Select, roasted	3 oz	137	0	0
eye of round, lean & fat, trim ¼ in, Select, roasted	3 oz	184	0	0
eye of round, lean & fat, trim ¼ in, Choice, roasted	3 oz	205	0	0
flank, lean & fat, trim 0 in, braised	3 oz	224	0	0
flank, lean & fat, trim 0 in, broiled	3 oz	192	0	0
porterhouse steak, lean & fat, trim ¼ in, Choice, broiled	3 oz	260	0	0
porterhouse steak, lean only, trim ¼ in, Choice, broiled	3 oz	185	0	0
rib eye small end, lean & fat, trim 0 in, Choice, broiled	3 oz	261	0	0
rib large end, lean & fat, trim 0 in, roasted	3 oz	300	0	0
rib large end, lean & fat, trim ¼ in, broiled	3 oz	295	0	0
rib large end, lean & fat, trim ¼ in, roasted	3 oz	310	0	0
rib small end, lean & fat, trim 0 in, broiled	3 oz	252	0	0
rib small end, lean & fat, trim ¼ in, broiled	3 oz	285	0	0
rib small end, lean & fat, trim ¼ in, roasted	3 oz	295	0	0
rib whole, lean & fat, trim ¼ in, Choice, broiled	3 oz	306	0	0
rib whole, lean & fat, trim ¼ in, Choice, roasted	3 oz	320	0	0

FOOD	PORTION	CAL	VIT A	VIT C
rib whole, lean & fat, trim ¼ in, Prime, roasted	3 oz	348	0	0
rib whole, lean & fat, trim ¼ in, Select, broiled	3 oz	274	0	0
rib whole, lean & fat, trim ¼ in, Select, roasted	3 oz	286	0	0
shank crosscut, lean & fat, trim ¼ in, Choice, simmered	3 oz	224	0	0
short loin top loin, lean & fat, trim 0 in, Choice, broiled	1 steak (5.4 oz)	353	0	0
short loin top loin, lean & fat, trim 0 in, Choice, broiled	3 oz	193	0	0
short loin top loin, lean & fat, trim 0 in, Select, broiled	1 steak (5.4 oz)	309	0	0
short loin top loin, lean & fat, trim ¼ in, Prime, broiled	1 steak (6.3 oz)	582	0	0
short loin top loin, lean & fat, trim ¼ in, Select, broiled	1 steak (6.3 oz)	473	0	0
short loin top loin, lean & fat, trim ¼ in, Choice, broiled	1 steak (6.3 oz)	536	0	0
short loin top loin, lean & fat, trim ¼ in, Choice, broiled	3 oz	253	0	0
short loin top loin, lean only, trim 0 in, Choice, broiled	1 steak (5.2 oz)	311	0	0
short loin top loin, lean only, trim ¼ in, Choice, broiled	1 steak (5.2 oz)	314	0	0
t-bone steak, lean & fat, trim ¼ in, Choice, broiled	3 oz	253	0	0
t-bone steak, lean only, trim ¼ in, Choice, broiled	3 oz	182	0	0
tenderloin, lean & fat, trim ¼ in, Choice, broiled	3 oz	259	0	0
tenderloin, lean & fat, trim ¼ in, Choice, roasted	3 oz	288	0	0
tenderloin, lean & fat, trim ¼ in, Prime, broiled	3 oz	270	0	0

FOOD	PORTION	CAL	VIT A	VIT C
tenderloin, lean & fat, trim ¼ in, Select, roasted	3 oz	275	0	0
tenderloin, lean & fat, trim 0 in, Select, broiled	3 oz	194	0	0
tenderloin, lean & fat, trim 0 in, Choice, broiled	3 oz	208	0	0
tenderloin, lean only, trim ¼ in, Choice, broiled	3 oz	188	0	0
tenderloin, lean only, trim ¼ in, Select, broiled	3 oz	169	0	0
tenderloin, lean only, trim 0 in, Select, broiled	3 oz	170	0	0
tip round, lean & fat, trim ¼ in, Choice, roasted	3 oz	210	0	0
tip round, lean & fat, trim ¼ in, Prime, roasted	3 oz	233	0	0
tip round, lean & fat, trim ¼ in, Select, roasted	3 oz	191	0	0
tip round, lean & fat, trim 0 in, Choice, roasted	3 oz	170	0	0
tip round, lean & fat, trim 0 in, Select, roasted	3 oz	158	0	0
top round, lean & fat, trim ¼ in, Choice, braised	3 oz	221	0	0
top round, lean & fat, trim ¼ in, Choice, broiled	3 oz	190	0	0
top round, lean & fat, trim ¼ in, Choice, fried	3 oz	235	0	0
top round, lean & fat, trim ¼ in, Prime, broiled	3 oz	195	0	0
top round, lean & fat, trim ¼ in, Select, braised	3 oz	175	0	0
top round, lean & fat, trim ¼ in, Select, braised	3 oz	199	0	0
top round, lean & fat, trim 0 in, Choice, braised	3 oz	184	0	0

FOOD	PORTION	CAL	VIT A	VIT C
top round, lean & fat, trim 0 in, Select, braised	3 oz	170	0	0
top sirloin, lean & fat, trim ¼ in, Choice, broiled	3 oz	228	0	0
top sirloin, lean & fat, trim ¼ in, Choice, fried	3 oz	277	0	0
top sirloin, lean & fat, trim ¼ in, Select, broiled	3 oz	208	0	0
top sirloin, lean & fat, trim 0 in, Choice, broiled	3 oz	194	0	0
top sirloin, lean & fat, trim 0 in, Select, broiled	3 oz	166	0	0
tripe, raw	4 oz	111	0	4

BEEF DISHES
(Some of the vitamin A in the beef dishes comes from non-plant sources.)

FOOD	PORTION	CAL	VIT A	VIT C
CANNED				
Beef Stew (Healthy Choice)	½ can (7.5 oz)	140	1500	4
Manwich Mexican, as prep	1 sandwich	310	200	3
Sloppy Joe, as prep (Manwich)	1 sandwich	310	91	3
MIX				
Hamburger Helper Hamburger Pizza Dish, as prep	1 cup	360	500	1
Lipton Microeasy Hearty Beef Stew	¼ pkg	71	2190	14
Lipton Microeasy Homestyle Meatloaf	¼ pkg	87	1274	17
Manwich Seasoning Mix, as prep	1 sandwich	320	200	3
SHELF STABLE				
Beef Stew (Healthy Choice)	7.5-oz cup	140	1500	4
TAKE-OUT				
bubble & squeak	5 oz	186	180	10

FOOD	PORTION	CAL	VIT A	VIT C
cornish pasty	1 (8 oz)	847	0	0
kebab, indian	1 (5.4 oz)	553	495	3
kheena	6.7 oz	781	780	2
koftas	5	280	250	2

BISCUIT

FOOD	PORTION	CAL	VIT A	VIT C
Hungry Jack				
Buttermilk Flaky	1	90	0	0
Buttermilk Fluffy	1	90	0	0
Extra Rich Buttermilk	1	50	0	0
Flaky	1	80	0	0
Honey Tastin' Flaky	1	90	0	0
Pillsbury				
Butter	1	50	0	0
Buttermilk	1	50	0	0
Country	1	50	0	0
Good 'N Buttery Fluffy	1	90	0	0
Heat N' Eat Big Premium	2	280	0	0
Tender Layer Buttermilk	1	50	0	0
Pillsbury Big Country Butter Tastin'	1	100	0	0
Pillsbury Big Country Buttermilk	1	100	0	0
Pillsbury Deluxe Heat N' Eat Buttermilk	2	170	0	0
buttermilk	1 (1 oz)	98	0	0
plain	1 (1 oz)	98	0	0
TAKE-OUT				
(Vitamin A in take-out biscuits comes from eggs, a non-plant source.)				
plain	1 (35 g)	276	98	0
w/ egg	1	315	649	0

FOOD	PORTION	CAL	VIT A	VIT C
w/ egg & bacon	1	457	191	3
w/ egg & sausage	1	582	635	tr
w/ egg & steak	1	474	704	tr
w/ egg, cheese & bacon	1	477	648	2
w/ ham	1	387	133	tr
w/ sausage	1	485	56	tr
w/ steak	1	456	65	tr

BLACK BEANS

CANNED

FOOD	PORTION	CAL	VIT A	VIT C
Health Valley Fast Menu Organic Black Beans With Tofu Wieners	7.5 oz	150	4184	tr
Health Valley Fast Menu Western Black Beans With Garden Vegetable	7.5 oz	160	5000	1

DRIED

FOOD	PORTION	CAL	VIT A	VIT C
cooked	1 cup	227	10	0

BLACKBERRIES

CANNED

FOOD	PORTION	CAL	VIT A	VIT C
in heavy syrup	½ cup	118	280	4

FRESH

FOOD	PORTION	CAL	VIT A	VIT C
blackberries	½ cup	37	119	15

FROZEN

FOOD	PORTION	CAL	VIT A	VIT C
unsweetened	1 cup	97	172	5

BLACKEYE PEAS

CANNED

FOOD	PORTION	CAL	VIT A	VIT C
Trappey's	½ cup	90	tr	tr
Trappey's Jalapeno	½ cup	90	tr	tr
w/ pork	½ cup	199	0	1

DRIED

FOOD	PORTION	CAL	VIT A	VIT C
cooked	1 cup	198	26	1

FOOD	PORTION	CAL	VIT A	VIT C
BLINTZE				
TAKE-OUT				
cheese	2	186	177	0
BLUEBERRIES				
CANNED				
In Heavy Syrup (S&W)	½ cup	111	200	24
in heavy syrup	1 cup	225	164	3
FRESH				
blueberries	1 cup	82	145	19
FROZEN				
unsweetened	1 cup	78	126	4
BLUEFIN				
(Vitamin A in bluefin comes from a non-plant source.)				
fillet, baked	4.1 oz	186	537	tr
BLUEFISH				
(Vitamin A in bluefish comes from a non-plant source.)				
FRESH				
baked	3 oz	135	390	tr
BOK CHOY				
Dole, shredded	½ cup	5	1050	16
BORAGE				
FRESH				
cooked, chopped	3.5 oz	25	4385	33
raw, chopped	½ cup	9	1848	15
BOYSENBERRIES				
CANNED				
in heavy syrup	1 cup	226	102	16
FROZEN				
unsweetened	1 cup	66	89	4

FOOD	PORTION	CAL	VIT A	VIT C

BRAINS

FOOD	PORTION	CAL	VIT A	VIT C
beef, pan-fried	3 oz	167	0	3
beef, simmered	3 oz	136	0	1
lamb, braised	3 oz	124	0	10
lamb, fried	3 oz	232	0	20
pork, braised	3 oz	117	0	12
veal, braised	3 oz	115	0	11
veal, fried	3 oz	181	0	12

BRAN

FOOD	PORTION	CAL	VIT A	VIT C
Fast Menu Oat Bran Pilaf With Garden Vegetables (Health Valley)	7.5 oz	210	6174	5
Oat Bran (Mother's)	⅓ cup	92	26	0
Quaker Unprocessed Bran	2 tbsp	8	0	0
Toasted Wheat Bran (Kretschmer)	⅓ cup	57	0	0
corn	⅓ cup	56	18	0

BRAZIL NUTS

FOOD	PORTION	CAL	VIT A	VIT C
dried, unblanched	1 oz	186	0	tr

BREAD
(Vitamin A in bread is usually from eggs and milk, non-plant sources; exception in this category are pumpkin, naan and paratha, rich in plant sources.)

FOOD	PORTION	CAL	VIT A	VIT C
CANNED				
boston brown	1 slice (1.6 oz)	88	39	0
HOME RECIPE				
banana	1 slice (2 oz)	195	278	1
cornbread, as prep w/ 2% milk	1 piece (2.3 oz)	173	180	tr
cornbread, as prep w/ whole milk	1 piece (2.3 oz)	176	158	tr

FOOD	PORTION	CAL	VIT A	VIT C
irish soda bread	1 slice (2 oz)	174	116	1
pumpkin	1 slice (1 oz)	94	1540	tr
white, as prep w/ 2% milk	1 slice	81	22	tr
white, as prep w/ nonfat dry milk	1 slice	78	12	0
white, as prep w/ whole milk	1 slice	82	14	tr
whole wheat	1 slice	79	0	0
MIX				
Corn Bread (Ballard)	⅛ bread	140	0	0
cornbread	1 piece (2 oz)	189	123	tr
READY-TO-EAT				
Fiber Calcium (Thomas')	1 slice	52	10	tr
Pita Wheat Mini (Sahara)	1 pocket (1 oz)	66	24	tr
Pita White (Sahara)	½ pocket	78	15	0
Pita White Mini (Sahara)	1 pocket	79	15	0
Wheat Lite (Thomas')	1 slice	41	13	tr
egg	1 slice (1.4 oz)	115	30	0
french	1 loaf (1 lb)	1270	tr	tr
french	1 slice (1 oz)	78	0	0
italian	1 loaf (1 lb)	1255	0	0
italian	1 slice (1 oz)	81	0	0
navajo fry	1 (10.5-in diam)	527	0	0
navajo fry	1 (5-in diam)	296	0	0
pita	1 reg (2 oz)	165	0	0
pita	1 sm (1 oz)	78	0	0
pita, whole wheat	1 reg (2 oz)	170	0	0
pita, whole wheat	1 sm (1 oz)	76	0	0
pumpernickel	1 slice	80	0	0
seven grain	1 slice	65	0	tr
sourdough	1 slice (1 oz)	78	0	0
vienna	1 slice (1 oz)	78	0	0

FOOD	PORTION	CAL	VIT A	VIT C
wheat berry	1 slice	65	0	0
white	1 slice	67	0	0
white, cubed	1 cup	80	tr	tr
white, toasted	1 slice	67	0	0
REFRIGERATED				
Pillsbury Crusty French Loaf	1-in slice	60	0	0
Pillsbury Pipin' Hot Wheat Loaf	1-in slice	70	0	0
Pillsbury Pipin' Hot White Loaf	1-in slice	70	0	0
TAKE-OUT				
chapatis, as prep w/o fat	1 (2.5 oz)	141	0	0
cornstick	1 (1.3 oz)	101	52	tr
naan	1 (6 oz)	571	825	tr
paratha	1 (4.4 oz)	403	875	0

BREAD COATING

Shake 'N Bake Original Barbecue For Chicken	¼ pkg (½ oz)	93	387	2
Shake 'N Bake Original Barbecue For Pork	¼ pkg (½ oz)	38	159	1
Shake 'N Bake Original Country Mild	¼ pkg (½ oz)	76	445	1

BREADCRUMBS

fresh	⅔	76	0	0

BREADFRUIT

fresh	¼ small	99	38	28
seeds, raw	1 oz	54	73	2

BREADSTICKS

Soft Bread Sticks (Pillsbury)	1	100	0	0
plain	1 sm	25	0	0

FOOD	PORTION	CAL	VIT A	VIT C
BREAKFAST BAR				
Apple (Nutri-Grain)	1 (1.3 oz)	150	750	tr
Blueberry (Nutri-Grain)	1 (1.3 oz)	150	750	tr
Raspberry (Nutri-Grain)	1 (1.3 oz)	150	750	tr
Strawberry (Nutri-Grain)	1 (1.3 oz)	150	750	tr

BREAKFAST DRINKS
(A portion of the vitamin A in breakfast drinks comes from milk, a non-plant source.)

FOOD	PORTION	CAL	VIT A	VIT C
Instant Breakfast Chocolate Malt, as prep w/ whole milk (Pillsbury)	1 serving	290	1500	18
Instant Breakfast Chocolate, as prep w/ whole milk (Pillsbury)	1 serving	290	1500	18
Instant Breakfast Strawberry, as prep w/ whole milk (Pillsbury)	1 serving	290	1500	18
Instant Breakfast Vanilla, as prep w/ whole milk (Pillsbury)	1 serving	300	1500	18
orange drink powder	3 rounded tsp	93	1490	98
orange drink powder, as prep w/ water	6 oz	86	1376	91

BROAD BEANS

FOOD	PORTION	CAL	VIT A	VIT C
CANNED				
broad beans	1 cup	183	26	5
DRIED				
cooked	1 cup	186	26	1
FRESH				
cooked	3.5 oz	56	270	20

BROCCOLI

FOOD	PORTION	CAL	VIT A	VIT C
Dole	1 med spear	40	721	139
chopped, cooked	½ cup	22	1082	58

FOOD	PORTION	CAL	VIT A	VIT C
raw, chopped	½ cup	12	678	41
FROZEN				
Baby Spears Deluxe (Birds Eye)	⅔ cup	30	1250	72
Big Valley	3.5 oz	25	1250	60
Broccoli With Cheese In Pastry (Pepperidge Farm)	1	230	400	12
Chopped (Birds Eye)	⅔ cup	25	2250	54
Cuts (Green Giant)	½ cup	12	400	30
Farm Fresh Spears (Birds Eye)	¾ cup	30	5500	66
Florets Deluxe (Birds Eye)	½ cup	25	1250	54
Harvest Fresh Cut (Green Giant)	½ cup	16	500	36
Harvest Fresh Spears (Green Giant)	½ cup	20	500	54
In Butter Sauce (Green Giant)	½ cup	40	1000	42
In Cheese Sauce (Green Giant)	½ cup	60	1000	36
Mini Spears Select (Green Giant)	4–5 spears	18	500	42
One Serve Cuts In Butter Sauce (Green Giant)	1 pkg	45	500	54
One Serve Cuts In Cheese Sauce (Green Giant)	1 pkg	70	1250	42
Polybag Cuts (Birds Eye)	½ cup	25	2000	54
Polybag Deluxe Florets (Birds Eye)	⅔ cup	25	1000	60
Spears (Birds Eye)	⅔ cup	25	1250	54
Valley Combinations Broccoli Fanfare (Green Giant)	½ cup	80	300	24
With Cheese Sauce (Birds Eye)	½ pkg	110	500	27
chopped, cooked	½ cup	25	1741	37
spears, cooked	½ cup	25	1741	37
spears, cooked	10-oz pkg	69	4730	100

FOOD	PORTION	CAL	VIT A	VIT C

BROWNIE

HOME RECIPE

FOOD	PORTION	CAL	VIT A	VIT C
w/ nuts	1 (0.8 oz)	95	20	tr

MIX

FOOD	PORTION	CAL	VIT A	VIT C
Deluxe Family-Size Fudge Brownie (Pillsbury)	2-in sq	150	0	0
Deluxe Fudge Brownie (Pillsbury)	2-in sq	150	0	0
Deluxe Fudge Brownie With Walnuts (Pillsbury)	2-in sq	150	0	0
Fudge Microwave (Pillsbury)	1	190	0	0
The Ultimate Carmel Fudge Chunk Brownie (Pillsbury)	2-in sq	170	0	0
The Ultimate Double Fudge Brownie (Pillsbury)	2-in sq	160	0	0
The Ultimate Rockey Road Fudge Brownie (Pillsbury)	2-in sq	170	0	0

READY-TO-EAT

FOOD	PORTION	CAL	VIT A	VIT C
w/ nuts	1 (1 oz)	100	70	tr
w/o nuts	1 (2 oz)	243	10	3

BRUSSELS SPROUTS

FRESH

FOOD	PORTION	CAL	VIT A	VIT C
Dole	½ cup	19	389	37
cooked	1 sprout	8	151	13
cooked	½ cup	30	561	48
raw	1 sprout	8	168	16
raw	½ cup	19	389	37

FROZEN

FOOD	PORTION	CAL	VIT A	VIT C
Birds Eye	½ cup	35	750	66
Green Giant	½ cup	25	0	5
In Butter Sauce (Green Giant)	½ cup	40	500	42
Whole (Big Valley)	3.5 oz	30	500	78
cooked	½ cup	33	459	36

FOOD	PORTION	CAL	VIT A	VIT C

BURDOCK ROOT

FRESH

raw	1 cup	85	0	4

BUTTER

clarified butter	3.5 oz	876	3750	0
regular butter	1 pat	36	153	0
regular butter	1 stick (4 oz)	813	3468	0
whipped butter	4 oz	542	2312	0

BUTTER BEANS

CANNED

| Trappey's Large White | ½ cup | 80 | 100 | tr |
| Van Camp's | 1 cup | 162 | 0 | 0 |

BUTTER BLENDS

(The vitamin A in butter blend comes from both animal and plant sources.)

| Le Slim Cow, soft | 1 tbsp | 40 | 1500 | 20 |
| regular butter blend | 1 stick | 811 | 3624 | tr |

BUTTERBUR

| canned fuki, chopped | 1 cup | 3 | 0 | 15 |
| fresh fuki, raw | 1 cup | 13 | 47 | 30 |

CABBAGE

Dole	½ med head	18	69	41
Dole Napa, shredded	½ cup	6	456	10
chinese pak-choi, raw, shredded	½ cup	5	1050	16
chinese pak-choi, shredded, cooked	½ cup	10	2183	22
chinese pe-tsai, raw, shredded	1 cup	12	912	21

FOOD	PORTION	CAL	VIT A	VIT C
chinese pe-tsai, shredded, cooked	1 cup	16	1151	19
danish, raw	1 head (2 lbs)	228	1210	292
danish, raw, shredded	½ cup (1.2 oz)	9	47	11
danish, shredded, cooked	½ cup (2.6 oz)	17	99	15
green, raw	1 head (2 lbs)	228	1210	292
green, raw, shredded	½ cup (1.2 oz)	9	47	11
green, shredded, cooked	½ cup (2.6 oz)	17	99	15
red, raw, shredded	½ cup	10	14	20
red, shredded, cooked	½ cup	16	20	26
savoy, raw, shredded	½ cup	10	350	11
savoy, shredded, cooked	½ cup	18	649	12
HOME RECIPE				
coleslaw w/ dressing	¾ cup	147	337	8
TAKE-OUT				
coleslaw w/ dressing	½ cup	42	381	20
stuffed cabbage	1 (6 oz)	373	776	7
sweet & sour red cabbage	4 oz	61	170	14
vinegar & oil coleslaw	3.5 oz	150	500	30

CAKE

(Vitamin A in cakes comes from non-plant ingredients; the exception is carrot cake.)

FROSTING/ICING
Pillsbury

FOOD	PORTION	CAL	VIT A	VIT C
Cake & Cookie Decorator Chocolate	1 tbsp	60	0	0
Cake & Cookie Decorator, all colors except chocolate	1 tbsp	70	0	0
Chocolate Fudge	⅙ cake	110	0	0
Coconut Almond Frosting Mix	1⁄12 cake	160	100	0

FOOD	PORTION	CAL	VIT A	VIT C
Fluffy White Frosting Mix	1/12 cake	60	0	0
Frost It Hot Chocolate	1/8 cake	50	0	0
Frost It Hot Fluffy White	1/8 cake	50	0	0
Frosting Supreme Caramel Pecan	1/12 cake	160	0	0
Frosting Supreme Chocolate Chip	1/12 cake	150	0	0
Frosting Supreme Chocolate Fudge	1/12 cake	150	0	0
Frosting Supreme Chocolate Mint	1/12 cake	150	0	0
Frosting Supreme Coconut Almond	1/12 cake	150	0	0
Frosting Supreme Coconut Pecan	1/12 cake	160	0	0
Frosting Supreme Cream Cheese	1/12 cake	160	0	0
Frosting Supreme Double Dutch	1/12 cake	140	0	0
Frosting Supreme Lemon	1/12 cake	160	0	0
Frosting Supreme Milk Chocolate	1/12 cake	150	0	0
Frosting Supreme Mocha	1/12 cake	150	0	0
Frosting Supreme Sour Cream Vanilla	1/12 cake	160	0	0
Frosting Supreme Strawberry	1/12 cake	160	0	0
Frosting Supreme Vanilla	1/12 cake	160	0	0
Funfetti Chocolate Fudge	1/12 can	140	0	0
Funfetti Vanilla Pink	1/12 can	150	0	0
Funfetti Vanilla White	1/12 can	150	0	0
Vanilla	1/8 can	120	0	0
FROZEN				
Apple Crisp Light (Sara Lee)	1 (3 oz)	150	200	1

FOOD	PORTION	CAL	VIT A	VIT C
Black Forest Light (Sara Lee)	1 (3.6 oz)	170	600	1
Carrot Classic (Pepperidge Farm)	1 cake	260	1000	1
Carrot Light (Sara Lee)	1 (2.5 oz)	170	1500	0
Cheesecake Original Strawberry (Sara Lee)	1 slice (3.2 oz)	222	200	5
Cheesecake Original Cherry (Sara Lee)	1 slice (3.2 oz)	243	400	9
Cheesecake Original Plain (Sara Lee)	1 slice (2.8 oz)	230	300	1
Cherries Supreme Dessert Lights (Pepperidge Farm)	1 piece (3.25 oz)	170	400	1
Chocolate Free & Light (Sara Lee)	1 slice (1.7 oz)	110	100	0
Double Chocolate Light (Sara Lee)	1 (2.5 oz)	150	300	0
French Cheesecake Light (Sara Lee)	1 (3.2 oz)	150	200	0
Lemon Cake Supreme Dessert Lights (Pepperidge Farm)	1 piece (2.75 oz)	170	100	9
Lemon Cream Light (Sara Lee)	1 (3.2 oz)	180	100	0
Peach Parfait Dessert Lights (Pepperidge Farm)	1 piece (4.25 oz)	150	300	24
Peach Turnover (Pepperidge Farm)	1	310	300	36
Strawberry French Cheesecake Light (Sara Lee)	1 (3.5 oz)	150	500	2
Strawberry Shortcake Dessert Lights (Pepperidge Farm)	1 piece (3 oz)	170	200	12
Strawberry Shortcake Two Layer (Sara Lee)	1 slice (2.5 oz)	190	100	4
Strawberry Yogurt Dessert Free & Light (Sara Lee)	1 slice (2.2 oz)	120	400	2
HOME RECIPE angelfood	½ cake (1.9 oz)	142	0	0

FOOD	PORTION	CAL	VIT A	VIT C
boston cream pie	⅙ cake (3.3 oz)	293	180	tr
carrot w/ cream cheese icing	1 cake (10-in diam)	6175	2240	23
carrot w/ cream cheese icing	1/12 cake (3.9 oz)	484	3827	1
chocolate w/o frosting	1/12 cake (3.3 oz)	340	133	tr
chocolate w/o frosting	2 layers (39.9 oz)	4067	1596	2
eclair	1 (3 oz)	262	718	tr
fruitcake	1/36 cake (2.9 oz)	302	60	4
fruitcake, dark	1 cake (7½ × 2¼ in)	5185	1720	504
gingerbread	⅑ cake (2.6 oz)	264	36	tr
pineapple upside down	⅑ cake (4 oz)	367	291	1
pound cake	1 loaf (8½ × 3½ in)	1935	3470	1
pound cake	1 slice (1 oz)	120	200	tr
sheet cake w/ white frosting	1 cake (9-in sq)	4020	2190	2
sheet cake w/ white frosting	⅑ cake	445	240	tr
sheet cake w/o frosting	1 cake (9-in sq)	2830	1320	2
sheet cake w/o frosting	⅑ cake	315	150	tr
shortcake	1 (2.3 oz)	225	47	tr
sponge cake	1/12 cake (2.2 oz)	140	121	0
white w/ coconut frosting	1/12 cake (3.9 oz)	399	43	tr
white w/o frosting	1/12 cake (2.6 oz)	264	42	tr
MIX				
Jell-O Cheesecake New York Style	⅙ cake	283	361	1
Pillsbury				
Apple Cinnamon Coffee Cake	⅛ cake	240	0	0
Banana Quick Bread	1/12 loaf	170	0	0
Blueberry Nut Quick Bread	1/12 loaf	150	0	0

FOOD	PORTION	CAL	VIT A	VIT C
Pillsbury (cont.)				
Butter Recipe	1/12 cake	260	300	0
Cherry Nut Quick Bread	1/12 loaf	180	0	0
Chocolate Microwave	1/8 cake	210	0	0
Chocolate Chip	1/12 cake	270	0	0
Chocolate With Chocolate Frosting	1/8 cake	300	0	0
Chocolate With Vanilla Frosting	1/8 cake	300	0	0
Cranberry Quick Bread	1/12 loaf	160	0	0
Date Quick Bread	1/12 loaf	160	0	0
Devil's Food	1/12 cake	270	0	0
Double Chocolate Supreme Microwave	1/8 cake	330	0	0
Double Lemon Supreme Microwave	1/8 cake	300	0	0
Fudge Marble	1/12 cake	270	100	0
Gingerbread	3-in sq	190	0	0
Lemon	1/12 cake	250	0	0
Lemon Microwave	1/8 cake	220	0	0
Lemon With Lemon Frosting	1/8 cake	300	0	0
Nut Quick Bread	1/12 loaf	170	0	0
Strawberry	1/12 cake	260	100	0
Streusel Swirl Cinnamon	1/16 cake	260	100	0
Streusel Swirl Cinnamon Microwave	1/8 cake	240	0	0
Streusel Swirl Lemon	1/16 cake	270	100	0
Tunnel Of Fudge Bundt Microwave	1/8 cake	290	0	0
White	1/12 cake	240	0	0
Yellow	1/12 cake	260	100	0

FOOD	PORTION	CAL	VIT A	VIT C
Yellow Microwave	⅛ cake	220	0	0
Yellow With Chocolate Frosting	⅛ cake	300	0	0
angelfood	1/12 cake (1.8 oz)	129	0	0
angelfood	10 in cake (20.9 oz)	1535	0	0
chocolate w/o frosting low sodium	1/10 cake (1.3 oz)	116	0	0
crumb coffeecake	1 cake (7¾ × 5⅝ in)	1385	690	1
crumb coffeecake	⅛ cake	230	120	tr
devil's food w/ chocolate frosting	1 cake (9-in diam)	3755	1660	1
devil's food w/ chocolate frosting	1/16 cake	235	100	tr
gingerbread	1 cake (8-in sq)	1575	0	1
lemon w/o frosting no sugar low sodium	1/10 cake (1.3 oz)	118	0	0
white w/o frosting no sugar low sodium	1/10 cake (1.3 oz)	118	0	0
yellow w/ chocolate frosting	1 cake (9-in diam)	3895	1850	0
READY-TO-EAT				
angelfood	1 cake (11.9 oz)	876	0	0
angelfood	1/12 cake (1 oz)	73	0	0
bakewell tart	1 slice (3 oz)	410	765	1
battenburg cake	1 slice (2 oz)	204	125	0
cheesecake	1 cake (9-in diam)	3350	2820	56
cheesecake	(1/12 cake)	280	230	5
cherry fudge w/ chocolate frosting	⅛ cake (2.5 oz)	187	158	10

FOOD	PORTION	CAL	VIT A	VIT C
crumpets, toasted	2 (4 oz)	119	0	0
eccles cake	1 slice (2 oz)	285	185	0
eclair	1 (1.4 oz)	149	420	tr
pound cake	1 cake (8½ × 3½ × 3 in)	1935	2820	0
pound cake	1 slice (1 oz)	110	160	0
sponge	½2 cake (1.3 oz)	110	59	0
strudel, apple	1 piece (2½ oz)	195	21	1
treacle tart	1 slice (2.5 oz)	258	210	0
vanilla slice	1 slice (2½ oz)	248	60	1
white w/ white frosting	1 cake (9 in diam)	4170	640	0
white w/ white frosting	½6 cake	260	40	0
yellow w/ chocolate frosting	1 cake (9 diam)	3895	1850	0
REFRIGERATED				
Apple Turnovers (Pillsbury)	1	170	0	0
Cherry Turnovers (Pillsbury)	1	170	0	4
Coffee Cake Cinnamon Swirl (Pillsbury)	⅛ cake	180	0	0
Coffee Cake Pecan Struesel (Pillsbury)	⅛ cake	180	0	0
Pastry Pockets (Pillsbury)	1	240	0	0
SNACK				
Coffee Cake (Drake's)	1 (1.1 oz)	140	tr	tr
Coffee Cake Apple Cinnamon (Sara Lee)	1	290	200	12
Coffee Cake Chocolate Crumb (Drake's)	1 (2.5 oz)	245	tr	tr
Coffee Cake Cinnamon Crumb (Drake's)	½2 cake (1.3 oz)	150	tr	tr

FOOD	PORTION	CAL	VIT A	VIT C
Coffee Cake Small (Drake's)	1 (2 oz)	220	tr	tr
Devil Dog (Drake's)	1 (1.5 oz)	160	tr	tr
Funny Bones (Drake's)	1 (1.25 oz)	150	tr	tr
Pop-Tarts				
Apple Cinnamon	1	210	500	tr
Blueberry	1	210	500	tr
Brown Sugar, Cinnamon	1	210	500	tr
Cherry	1	210	500	tr
Chocolate Graham	1	210	500	tr
Frosted Brown Sugar Cinnamon	1	210	500	tr
Frosted Cherry	1	210	500	tr
Frosted Chocolate Vanilla Creme	1	200	500	tr
Frosted Chocolate Fudge	1	200	500	tr
Frosted Grape	1	200	500	tr
Frosted Raspberry	1	200	500	tr
Frosted Strawberry	1	200	500	tr
Strawberry	1	210	500	tr
Pound Cake (Drake's)	1	110	tr	tr
Ring Ding (Drake's)	1 (1.5 oz)	180	tr	tr
Ring Ding Mint (Drake's)	1 (1.5 oz)	190	tr	tr
Sunny Doodle (Drake's)	1 (1 oz)	100	tr	tr
Toast-R-Cakes BlueBerry	1	110	105	tr
Toast-R-Cakes Bran	1	103	59	tr
Toast-R-Cakes Corn	1	120	32	tr
Yankee Doodle (Drake's)	1 (1 oz)	100	tr	tr
Yodel's (Drake's)	1 (1 oz)	150	tr	tr
devil's food cupcake w/ chocolate frosting	1	120	50	tr
devil's food w/ creme filling	1 (1 oz)	105	20	0

FOOD	PORTION	CAL	VIT A	VIT C
TAKE-OUT				
baklava	1 oz	126	219	1
strudel	1 piece (4.1 oz)	272	322	4
trifle w/ cream	6 oz	291	665	7

CANADIAN BACON

unheated	2 slices (1.9 oz)	89	0	12

CANDY

Milky Way II (Mars)	1 bar (2 oz)	193	47	tr
boiled sweets	¼ lb	327	0	0
candied cherries	1 (4 g)	12	7	0
candied pineapple slice	1 slice (2 oz)	179	59	13
candy corn	1 oz	105	0	0
caramels, chocolate	1 oz	115	tr	tr
caramels, plain	1 oz	115	tr	tr
chocolate	1 oz	145	30	tr
chocolate crisp	1 oz	140	30	tr
chocolate w/ almonds	1 oz	150	30	tr
chocolate w/ peanuts	1 oz	155	30	tr
dark chocolate	1 oz	150	10	tr
fruit pastilles	1 tube (1.4 oz)	101	0	0
fudge, chocolate	1 oz	115	tr	tr
fudge, vanilla	1 oz	115	tr	tr
gum drops	1 oz	100	0	0
hard candy	1 oz	110	0	0
jelly beans	1 oz	105	0	0
mint fondant	1 oz	105	0	0

CANTALOUPE

Dole	¼	50	6382	63

FOOD	PORTION	CAL	VIT A	VIT C
cubed	1 cup	57	5158	68
half	½	94	8608	113

CARAMBOLA

fresh	1	42	626	27

CARDOON

fresh, cooked	3½ oz	22	118	2
raw, shedded	½ cup	36	107	2

CARISSA

fresh	1	12	8	8

CAROB

carob mix, as prep w/ whole milk	9 oz	195	307	2
flour	1 cup	185	15	tr
flour	1 tbsp	14	1	0

CARP

FRESH
cooked	1 fillet (6 oz)	276	54	3
cooked	3 oz	138	27	1
raw	3 oz	108	25	1

CARROTS

CANNED
Diced Fancy (S&W)	½ cup	30	3000	2
Julienne French Style Fancy (S&W)	½ cup	30	3000	2
Sliced Fancy (S&W)	½ cup	30	3000	2
Sliced Water Pack (S&W)	½ cup	30	12500	1

FOOD	PORTION	CAL	VIT A	VIT C
Whole Tiny Fancy (S&W)	½ cup	30	3000	2
slices	½ cup	17	10055	2
slices low sodium	½ cup	17	10055	2
FRESH				
Dole	1 med	40	16065	6
baby, raw	1 (½ oz)	6	296	1
raw	1 (2.5 oz)	31	20253	7
raw, shredded	½ cup	24	15471	5
slices, cooked	½ cup	35	19152	2
FROZEN				
Baby Whole Deluxe (Birds Eye)	½ cup	40	15000	6
Crinkle Cut (Big Valley)	3.5 oz	40	15000	5
Harvest Fresh Baby (Green Giant)	½ cup	18	9500	1
Polybag Sliced (Birds Eye)	¾ cup	35	15000	5
Whole (Big Valley)	3.5 oz	40	15000	5
slices, cooked	½ cup	26	12922	2
JUICE				
canned	6 oz	73	47381	16

CASABA

cubed	1 cup	45	51	27
fresh	⅒	43	49	26

CASHEWS

cashew butter w/o salt	1 tbsp	94	0	0
dry roasted	1 oz	163	0	0
dry roasted, salted	1 oz	163	0	0
oil roasted	1 oz	163	0	0
oil roasted, salted	1 oz	163	0	0

FOOD	PORTION	CAL	VIT A	VIT C

CASSAVA

raw	3½ oz	120	10	48

CATSUP

Hunt's	1 tbsp	15	17	17
Hunt's No Salt Added	1 tbsp	20	16	2
catsup	1 pkg (0.2 oz)	6	61	1
catsup	1 tbsp	16	152	2
low sodium	1 tbsp	16	152	2

CAULIFLOWER

FRESH

Dole	⅙ med head	18	17	53
cooked	½ cup (2.2 oz)	14	19	28
flowerets, cooked	3 (2 oz)	12	9	24
flowerets, raw	3 (2 oz)	14	11	26
raw	½ cup (1.8 oz)	13	10	23

FROZEN

Cuts (Green Giant)	½ cup	12	0	24
In Cheese Sauce (Green Giant)	½ cup	60	300	30
One Serve in Cheese Sauce (Green Giant)	1 pkg	80	400	42
Polybag (Birds Eye)	½ cup	20	3	48
With Cheddar Cheese Sauce (Budget Gourmet)	1 pkg	130	400	18
cooked	½ cup	17	20	28

CELERIAC

fresh, cooked	3½ oz	25	0	4
raw	½ cup	31	0	6

FOOD	PORTION	CAL	VIT A	VIT C

CELERY

FRESH
Dole	2 med stalks	20	156	9
diced, cooked	½ cup	13	99	5
raw	1 stalk (1.3 oz)	6	54	3
raw diced	½ cup	10	80	4

CELTUCE

raw	3½ oz	22	3500	20

CEREAL

COOKED
Enriched White Hominy Grits Quick (Quaker)	3 tbsp	101	0	0
Enriched White Hominy Grits Regular (Aunt Jemima)	3 tbsp	101	0	0
Enriched Yellow Hominy Quick Grits (Quaker)	3 tbsp	101	0	0
Farina (Pillsbury)	⅔ cup	80	0	0
Instant Grits White Hominy (Quaker)	1 pkg	79	0	0
Instant Grits With Imitation Bacon Bits (Quaker)	1 pkg	101	0	0
Instant Grits With Imitation Ham Bits (Quaker)	1 pkg	99	0	0
Instant Grits With Real Cheddar Cheese (Quaker)	1 pkg	104	400	0
Maypo 30 Second	1 oz	100	1500	18
Maypo (Vermont Style)	1 oz	105	1500	18
Maypo With Oat Bran	1 oz	130	2000	24
Oat Bran (Quaker)	⅓ cup	92	26	0
Oat Bran Natural Apples & Cinnamon (Health Valley)	¼ cup (1 oz)	100	tr	tr

FOOD	PORTION	CAL	VIT A	VIT C
Oat Bran Natural Raisins & Spice (Health Valley)	¼ cup	100	tr	1
Quaker				
Oatmeal Instant Apples & Cinnamon	1 pkg	118	1233	tr
Oatmeal Instant Cinnamon & Spice	1 pkg	164	1309	0
Oatmeal Instant Extra Fortified Apples & Spice	1 pkg	133	5001	60
Oatmeal Instant Extra Fortified Raisins & Cinnamon	1 pkg	129	5001	60
Oatmeal Instant Extra Fortified Regular	1 pkg	95	5115	60
Oatmeal Instant Maple & Brown Sugar	1 pkg	152	1380	0
Oatmeal Instant Peaches & Cream Flavors	1 pkg	129	1245	0
Oatmeal Instant Raisin & Spice	1 pkg	149	1298	0
Oatmeal Instant Raisin, Dates & Walnuts	1 pkg	141	988	0
Oatmeal Instant Regular	1 pkg	94	1237	0
Oatmeal Instant Strawberries & Cream Flavors	1 pkg	129	1186	0
Oats Old Fashion	⅔ cup	99	26	0
Oats Quick	⅔ cup	99	26	0
Whole Wheat Hot Natural Cereal	⅔ cup	92	26	0
oatmeal instant, cooked w/o salt	1 cup	145	40	0
oatmeal quick, cooked w/o salt	1 cup	145	40	0
oatmeal regular, cooked w/o salt	1 cup	145	40	0

FOOD	PORTION	CAL	VIT A	VIT C
READY-TO-EAT				
100% Natural Bran With Apples & Cinnamon (Health Valley)	¼ cup (1 oz)	100	tr	1
All-Bran (Kellogg's)	⅓ cup (1 oz)	70	750	15
All-Bran With Extra Fiber (Kellogg's)	½ cup (1 oz)	50	750	15
Apple Cinnamon Squares (Kellogg's)	½ cup (1 oz)	90	0	tr
Apple Jacks (Kellogg's)	1 cup (1 oz)	110	750	15
Apple Raisin Crisp (Kellogg's)	⅔ cup (1 oz)	130	750	tr
Basic 4 (General Mills)	¾ cup	130	1250	15
Blue Corn Flakes 100% Organic (Health Valley)	½ cup (1 oz)	90	203	0
Blueberry Squares (Kellogg's)	½ cup (1 oz)	90	0	tr
Body Buddies Natural Fruit (General Mills)	1 cup (1 oz)	110	1250	15
Booberry (General Mills)	1 cup (1 oz)	110	1250	12
Bran Buds (Kellogg's)	⅓ cup (1 oz)	70	750	15
Bran Cereal With Dates 100% Organic (Health Valley)	¼ cup (1 oz)	100	0	1
Bran Cereal With Raisins 100% Organic (Health Valley)	¼ cup (1 oz)	100	0	1
Bran Flakes (Kellogg's)	⅔ cup (1 oz)	90	750	tr
Cap'n Crunch (Quaker)	¾ cup	113	0	0
Cap'n Crunch's Crunchberries (Quaker)	¾ cup	113	0	0
Cap'n Crunch's Peanut Butter Crunch (Quaker)	¾ cup	119	0	0
Cheerios (General Mills)	1¼ cup (1 oz)	110	1250	15
Cheerios Apple Cinnamon (General Mills)	¾ cup (1 oz)	110	1250	15
Cheerios Honey Nut (General Mills)	¾ cup (1 oz)	110	1250	15

FOOD	PORTION	CAL	VIT A	VIT C
Cheerios-to-Go (General Mills)	1 pkg (0.75 oz)	80	750	9
Cheerios-to-Go Apple Cinnamon (General Mills)	1 pkg (1 oz)	110	1250	15
Cheerios-to-Go Honey Nut (General Mills)	1 pkg (1 oz)	110	1250	15
Cinnamon Mini Buns (Kellogg's)	¾ cup (1 oz)	110	750	15
Cinnamon Toast Crunch (General Mills)	¾ cup (1 oz)	120	1250	15
Clusters (General Mills)	½ cup (1 oz)	110	1250	15
Cocoa Krispies (Kellogg's)	¾ cup (1 oz)	110	750	15
Cocoa Puffs (General Mills)	1 cup (1 oz)	110	1250	15
Common Sense Oat Bran (Kellogg's)	¾ cup (1 oz)	100	750	tr
Common Sense Oat Bran With Raisins (Kellogg's)	¾ cup (1 oz)	130	750	tr
Corn Flakes (Kellogg's)	1 cup (1 oz)	100	750	15
Corn Pops (Kellogg's)	1 cup (1 oz)	110	750	15
Count Chocula (General Mills)	1 cup (1 oz)	110	1250	15
Country Corn Flakes (General Mills)	1 cup (1 oz)	110	1250	15
Cracklin' Oat Bran (Kellogg's)	½ cup (1 oz)	110	750	15
Crispix (Kellogg's)	1 cup (1 oz)	110	750	15
Crispy Wheats 'N Raisins (General Mills)	¾ cup (1 oz)	100	1250	15
Crunchy Bran (Quaker)	⅔ cup	89	0	0
Crunchy Nut Oh!s (Quaker)	1 cup	127	0	0
Double Dip Crunch (Kellogg's)	⅔ cup (1 oz)	120	750	15
Fiber 7 Flakes 100% Organic (Health Valley)	½ cup (1 oz)	90	73	1
Fiber 7 Flakes With Raisins 100% Organic (Health Valley)	½ cup (1 oz)	90	73	1
Fiber One (General Mills)	½ cup (1 oz)	60	1250	15

FOOD	PORTION	CAL	VIT A	VIT C
Fiberwise (Kellogg's)	⅔ cup (1 oz)	90	750	15
Frankenberry (General Mills)	1 cup (1 oz)	110	1250	15
Froot Loops (Kellogg's)	1 cup (1 oz)	110	750	60
Frosted Mini-Wheats (Kellogg's)	4 biscuits (1 oz)	100	0	tr
Frosted Mini-Wheats Bite Size (Kellogg's)	½ cup	100	0	tr
Frosted Bran (Kellogg's)	1.5 oz	150	1000	21
Frosted Flakes (Kellogg's)	¾ cup (1 oz)	110	750	15
Frosted Krispies (Kellogg's)	¾ cup (1 oz)	110	750	15
Fruit Lites Wheat (Health Valley)	½ cup (0.5 oz)	45	1	tr
Fruit Lites Corn (Health Valley)	½ cup (0.5 oz)	45	40	tr
Fruit Lites Rice (Health Valley)	½ cup (0.5 oz)	45	1	1
Fruitful Bran (Kellogg's)	⅔ cup (1.4 oz)	120	750	tr
Fruity Marshmallow Krispies (Kellogg's)	1¼ cups (1.3 oz)	140	750	15
Fruity Yummy Mummy (General Mills)	1 cup (1 oz)	110	1250	15
Golden Grahams (General Mills)	¾ cup (1 oz)	110	1250	15
Healthy Crunch Almond Date (Health Valley)	¼ cup (1 oz)	110	1	3
Healthy Crunch Apple Cinnamon (Health Valley)	¼ cup (1 oz)	110	tr	3
Healthy O's 100% Organic (Health Valley)	¾ cup (1 oz)	90	1	1
Honey Graham Oh!s (Quaker)	1 cup	122	0	0
Just Right With Fiber Nuggets (Kellogg's)	⅔ cup (1 oz)	100	5000	tr
Just Right With Raisins, Dates & Nuts (Kellogg's)	¾ cup (1.3 oz)	140	5000	tr
Kaboom (General Mills)	1 cup (1 oz)	110	2250	27

FOOD	PORTION	CAL	VIT A	VIT C
Kenmei (Kellogg's)	¾ cup (1 oz)	110	750	tr
King Vitamin (Quaker)	1½ cup	110	1500	24
Kix (General Mills)	1½ cup (1 oz)	110	1250	15
Life (Quaker)	⅔ cup	101	0	0
Life Cinnamon (Quaker)	⅔ cup	101	0	0
Lites Puffed Corn (Health Valley)	½ cup (1 oz)	50	72	tr
Lites Puffed Rice (Health Valley)	½ cup (1 oz)	50	0	1
Lites Puffed Wheat (Health Valley)	½ cup (1 oz)	50	0	1
Lucky Charms (General Mills)	1 cup (1 oz)	110	1250	15
Mueslix Crispy Blend (Kellogg's)	⅔ cup (1.5 oz)	150	750	tr
Mueslix Golden Crunch (Kellogg's)	½ cup (1.2 oz)	120	750	tr
Nut & Honey Crunch (Kellogg's)	⅔ cup (1 oz)	110	750	15
Nut & Honey Crunch O's (Kellogg's)	⅔ cup (1 oz)	110	750	15
Nutri-Grain Almond Raisin (Kellogg's)	⅔ cup (1.4 oz)	140	0	tr
Nutri-Grain Raisin Bran (Kellogg's)	1 cup (1.4 oz)	130	0	tr
Nutri-Grain Wheat (Kellogg's)	⅔ cup (1 oz)	90	0	15
Oat Bran Flakes 100% Organic (Health Valley)	½ cup (1 oz)	100	5	tr
Oat Bran Flakes Almonds/ Dates 100% Organic (Health Valley)	½ cup (1 oz)	100	8	tr
Oat Bran Flakes With Raisins 100% Organic (Health Valley)	½ cup (1 oz)	100	8	tr
Oat Bran O's 100% Organic (Health Valley)	½ cup (1 oz)	110	10	1

FOOD	PORTION	CAL	VIT A	VIT C
Oat Bran O's Fruit & Nuts (Health Valley)	½ cup (1 oz)	110	40	1
Oat Squares (Quaker)	½ cup	105	1616	0
Oatbake Honey Bran (Kellogg's)	⅓ cup (1 oz)	110	750	15
Oatbake Raisin Nut (Kellogg's)	⅓ cup (1 oz)	110	750	15
Oatmeal Crisp (General Mills)	½ cup (1 oz)	110	1250	15
Orangeola Almonds & Dates (Health Valley)	¼ cup	110	3	2
Orangeola Bananas & Hawaiian Fruit (Health Valley)	¼ cup (1 oz)	120	200	2
Popeye Sweet Crunch (Quaker)	1 cup	113	0	0
Product 19 (Kellogg's)	1 cup (1 oz)	100	750	60
Puffed Rice (Quaker)	1 cup	50	0	0
Puffed Wheat (Quaker)	1 cup	50	0	0
Quaker 100% Natural	¼ cup	127	0	0
Quaker 100% Natural Apples & Cinnamon	¼ cup	126	0	0
Quaker 100% Natural Raisins & Date	¼ cup	123	0	0
Raisin Bran (Kellogg's)	¾ cup (1.4 oz)	120	750	tr
Raisin Bran Flakes 100% Organic (Health Valley)	½ cup (1 oz)	100	tr	1
Raisin Nut Bran (General Mills)	½ cup (1 oz)	110	1250	15
Raisin Squares (Kellogg's)	½ cup (1 oz)	90	0	tr
Real Oat Bran Almond Crunch (Health Valley)	¼ cup (1 oz)	110	277	2
Real Oat Bran Hawaiian Fruit (Health Valley)	¼ cup (1 oz)	130	494	2
Real Oat Bran Raisin Nut (Health Valley)	¼ cup (1 oz)	130	144	2
Rice Bran O's (Health Valley)	½ cup	110	8	1

FOOD	PORTION	CAL	VIT A	VIT C
Rice Bran w/ Almonds & Dates (Health Valley)	½ cup (1 oz)	110	4	2
Rice Krispies (Kellogg's)	1 cup (1 oz)	110	750	15
S'Mores Grahams (General Mills)	¾ cup (1 oz)	120	1250	15
Shredded Wheat (Quaker)	2 biscuits	132	0	0
Special K (Kellogg's)	1 cup (1 oz)	100	750	15
Sprouts 7 Bananas & Hawaiian Fruit (Health Valley)	¼ cup (1 oz)	90	65	1
Sprouts 7 Raisin (Health Valley)	¼ cup	90	97	1
Strawberry Squares (Kellogg's)	½ cup (1 oz)	90	0	tr
Swiss Breakfast Raisin Nut (Health Valley)	¼ cup (1 oz)	100	1	1
Swiss Breakfast Tropical Fruit (Health Valley)	¼ cup (1 oz)	100	2	1
Team (Nabisco)	1 cup	110	1250	15
Total (General Mills)	1 cup (1 oz)	100	5000	60
Total Corn Flakes (General Mills)	1 cup (1 oz)	110	5000	60
Total Raisin Bran (General Mills)	1 cup (1.5 oz)	140	5000	60
Triples (General Mills)	¾ cup (1 oz)	110	1250	15
Trix (General Mills)	1 cup (1 oz)	110	1250	15
Weetabix	2 (1.3 oz)	142	0	0
Wheaties (General Mills)	1 cup (1 oz)	100	1250	15
Whole Grain Shredded Wheat (Kellogg's)	½ cup (1 oz)	90	0	tr
bran flakes	¾ cup (1 oz)	90	1250	0
corn flakes	1¼ cup (1 oz)	110	1250	15
granola	¼ cup	138	10	0
sugar-coated corn flakes	¾ cup (1 oz)	110	1250	15

FOOD	PORTION	CAL	VIT A	VIT C
CHAYOTE				
fresh, cooked	1 cup	38	75	13
raw	1 (7 oz)	49	114	22
raw, cut up	1 cup	32	74	15
CHEESE				
(The vitamin A in cheese comes from non-plant sources.)				
NATURAL				
Blue (Sargento)	1 oz	100	4	0
Brie (Sargento)	1 oz	95	4	0
Burger Cheese (Sargento)	1 oz	106	7	0
Cajun (Sargento)	1 oz	110	6	0
Camembert (Sargento)	1 oz	85	5	0
Cheddar (Sargento)	1 oz	114	6	0
Cheddar New York (Sargento)	1 oz	114	300	0
Cheddar Sharp Nut Log (Sargento)	1 oz	97	920	0
Colby (Sargento)	1 oz	112	293	0
Colby-Jack (Sargento)	1 oz	109	281	0
Edam (Sargento)	1 oz	101	260	0
Finland Swiss (Sargento)	1 oz	107	240	0
Fontina (Sargento)	1 oz	110	330	0
Fruit Moos Apricot (Dannon)	3.5 oz	150	400	0
Fruit Moos Banana (Dannon)	3.5 oz	150	400	0
Fruit Moos Raspberry (Dannon)	3.5 oz	150	400	0
Fruit Moos Strawberry (Dannon)	3.5 oz	150	400	0
Gouda (Sargento)	1 oz	101	183	0
Havarti (Sargento)	1 oz	118	231	0
Italian Style Grated Cheeses (Sargento)	1 oz	108	233	0

FOOD	PORTION	CAL	VIT A	VIT C
Limburger (Sargento)	1 oz	93	363	0
Monterey Jack (Sargento)	1 oz	106	269	0
Mozzarella Low Moisture Part Skim (Sargento)	1 oz	79	178	0
Mozzarella Whole Milk (Sargento)	1 oz	90	256	0
Muenster Red Rind (Sargento)	1 oz	104	318	0
Parmesan & Romano Grated (Sargento)	1 oz	111	167	0
Parmesan Fresh (Sargento)	1 oz	111	171	0
Parmesan Grated (Sargento)	1 oz	129	199	0
Port Wine Nut Log (Sargento)	1 oz	97	920	0
Provolone (Sargento)	1 oz	100	231	0
Queso Blanco (Sargento)	1 oz	104	318	0
Queso de Papa (Sargento)	1 oz	114	300	0
Ricotta Lite (Sargento)	1 oz	24	106	tr
Romano (Sargento)	1 oz	110	162	0
Smokestick (Sargento)	1 oz	103	229	0
String (Sargento)	1 oz	79	178	0
String Smoked (Sargento)	1 oz	79	178	0
Swiss (Sargento)	1 oz	107	240	0
Swiss Almond Nut Log (Sargento)	1 oz	94	920	0
Taco (Sargento)	1 oz	109	281	0
Tilsiter (Sargento)	1 oz	96	296	0
Tybo Red Wax (Sargento)	1 oz	98	215	0
blue	1 oz	100	204	0
blue, crumbled	1 cup	477	973	0
brick	1 oz	105	307	0
brie	1 oz	95	189	0
caerphilly	1.4 oz	150	700	tr

FOOD	PORTION	CAL	VIT A	VIT C
camembert	1 oz	85	262	0
camembert	1 wedge (1⅓ oz)	114	351	0
caraway	1 oz	107	299	0
cheddar	1 oz	114	300	0
cheddar, reduced fat	1.4 oz	104	365	tr
cheddar, shredded	1 cup	455	1197	0
cheshire	1 oz	110	279	0
cheshire, reduced fat	1.4 oz	108	325	tr
colby	1 oz	112	293	0
derby	1.4 oz	161	755	tr
double gloucester	1.4 oz	162	755	tr
edam	1 oz	101	260	0
edam, reduced fat	1.4 oz	92	170	tr
fontina	1 oz	110	333	0
fromage frais	1.6 oz	51	225	tr
gouda	1 oz	101	183	0
gruyere	1 oz	117	346	0
lancashire	1.4 oz	149	720	tr
leicester	1.4 oz	160	730	tr
limburger	1 oz	93	363	0
lymeswold	1.4 oz	170	990	tr
monterey	1 oz	106	269	0
mozzarella	1 lb	1276	3593	0
mozzarella	1 oz	80	225	0
mozzarella, low moisture	1 oz	90	256	0
mozzarella, low moisture part skim	1 oz	79	178	0
mozzarella, part skim	1 oz	72	166	0
muenster	1 oz	104	318	0
parmesan, grated	1 oz	129	199	0

FOOD	PORTION	CAL	VIT A	VIT C
parmesan, grated	1 tbsp	23	35	0
parmesan, hard	1 oz	111	171	0
port du salut	1 oz	100	378	0
provolone	1 oz	100	231	0
ricotta	1 cup	428	1205	0
ricotta	½ cup	216	608	0
ricotta, part skim	1 cup	340	1063	0
ricotta, part skim	½ cup	171	536	0
romano	1 oz	110	162	0
roquefort	1 oz	105	297	0
stilton, blue	1.4 oz	164	770	tr
stilton, white	1.4 oz	145	685	tr
swiss	1 oz	107	240	0
tilsit	1 oz	96	296	0
wensleydale	1.4 oz	151	635	tr
PROCESSED				
Kraft Pineapple Spread	1 oz	70	200	1
Lactaid American	3.5 oz	328	913	0
Sargento American Hot Pepper	1 oz	106	343	0
Sargento American Sharp Spread	1 oz	106	343	0
Sargento Imitation Mozzarella	1 oz	80	300	0
Sargento Brick	1 oz	95	325	0
Sargento Swiss	1 oz	95	229	0
american	1 oz	93	259	0
american cheese food	1 pkg (8 oz)	745	2073	0
american cheese spread	1 jar (5 oz)	412	1119	0
american cheese spread	1 oz	82	223	0
american cold pack	1 pkg (8 oz)	752	1600	0
swiss	1 oz	95	229	0
swiss cheese food	1 pkg (8 oz)	734	1943	0

FOOD	PORTION	CAL	VIT A	VIT C

CHEESE DISHES

HOME RECIPE

| welsh rarebit, as prep w/ 1 white toast | 1 slice | 228 | 825 | tr |

TAKE-OUT

cheese omelette, as prep w/ 2 eggs	1 (6.8 oz)	519	2750	tr
fondue	½ cup	303	692	tr
macaroni & cheese	6.3 oz	320	1100	tr

CHEESE SUBSTITUTES

| mozzarella | 1 oz | 70 | 413 | 0 |

CHERIMOYA

| fresh | 1 | 515 | 55 | 49 |

CHERRIES

CANNED

sour in heavy syrup	½ cup	232	1827	5
sour in water pack	1 cup	87	1840	5
sweet in heavy syrup	½ cup	107	199	5
sweet in juice pack	½ cup	68	156	3
sweet in light syrup	½ cup	85	197	5
sweet in water pack	½ cup	57	198	3

FRESH

Dole	1 cup	90	64	11
sour	1 cup	51	1321	10
sweet	10	49	146	5

FROZEN

Dark Sweet (Big Valley)	4 oz	60	100	9
sour, unsweetened	1 cup	72	1349	3
sweet, sweetened	1 cup	232	489	3

FOOD	PORTION	CAL	VIT A	VIT C
JUICE				
Dole Pure & Light	6 oz	90	33	2
Kool-Aid Koolers	1 (8.45 oz)	142	1	6
Smucker's Black Cherry	8 oz	130	100	4
Tang Fruit Box	8.45 oz	121	4	60
Wylers Drink Mix Wild Cherry	8 oz	81	0	11

CHESTNUTS

chinese, raw	1 oz	64	57	10
japanese, dried	1 oz	102	24	17
japanese, raw	1 oz	44	10	8
japanese, roasted	1 oz	57	21	8
roasted	1 cup	350	35	37
roasted	1 oz	70	7	7

CHICKEN
(The vitamin A in chicken comes from non-plant sources.)

FOOD	PORTION	CAL	VIT A	VIT C
CANNED				
chicken spread, barbeque flavored	1 oz	55	373	1
FRESH				
broiler/fryer				
back w/ skin, batter dipped & fried	½ back (2.5 oz)	238	85	0
back w/ skin, floured & fried	1.5 oz	146	54	0
back w/ skin, roasted	1 oz	96	111	0
back w/ skin, stewed	½ back (2.1 oz)	158	188	0
back w/o skin, fried	½ back (2 oz)	167	57	0
breast w/ skin, batter dipped & fried	½ breast (4.9 oz)	364	94	0
breast w/ skin, batter dipped & fried	2.9 oz	218	56	0
breast w/ skin, roasted	½ breast (3.4 oz)	193	91	0

FOOD	PORTION	CAL	VIT A	VIT C
Fresh broiler/fryer *(cont.)*				
breast w/ skin, roasted	2 oz	115	54	0
breast w/ skin, stewed	½ breast (3.9 oz)	202	90	0
breast w/o skin, fried	½ breast (3 oz)	161	20	0
breast w/o skin, roasted	½ breast (3 oz)	142	18	0
breast w/o skin, stewed	2 oz	86	11	0
dark meat w/ skin, batter dipped & fried	5.9 oz	497	172	0
dark meat w/ skin, floured & fried	3.9 oz	313	114	0
dark meat w/ skin, roasted	3.5 oz	256	203	0
dark meat w/ skin, stewed	3.9 oz	256	205	0
dark meat w/o skin, fried	1 cup (5 oz)	334	110	0
dark meat w/o skin, roasted	1 cup (5 oz)	286	101	0
dark meat w/o skin, stewed	1 cup (5 oz)	269	97	0
dark meat w/o skin, stewed	3 oz	165	59	0
drumstick w/ skin, batter dipped & fried	1 (2.6 oz)	193	62	0
drumstick w/ skin, floured & fried	1 (1.7 oz)	120	41	0
drumstick w/ skin, roasted	1 (1.8 oz)	112	52	0
drumstick w/ skin, stewed	1 (2 oz)	116	52	0
drumstick w/o skin, fried	1 (1.5 oz)	82	26	0
drumstick w/o skin, roasted	1 (1.5 oz)	76	26	0
drumstick w/o skin, stewed	1 (1.6 oz)	78	26	0
leg w/ skin, batter dipped & fried	1 (5.5 oz)	431	144	0
leg w/ skin, floured & fried	1 (3.9 oz)	285	103	0
leg w/ skin, roasted	1 (4 oz)	265	154	0
leg w/ skin, stewed	1 (4.4 oz)	275	156	0
leg w/o skin, fried	1 (3.3 oz)	195	62	0
leg w/o skin, roasted	1 (3.3 oz)	182	60	0
leg w/o skin, stewed	1 (3.5 oz)	187	60	0
light meat w/ skin, batter dipped & fried	4 oz	312	89	0
light meat w/ skin, floured & fried	2.7 oz	192	53	0
light meat w/ skin, roasted	2.8 oz	175	87	0
light meat w/ skin, stewed	3.2 oz	181	86	0
light meat w/o skin, fried	1 cup (5 oz)	268	42	0
light meat w/o skin, roasted	1 cup (5 oz)	242	41	0
light meat w/o skin, stewed	1 cup (5 oz)	223	37	0
neck w/ skin, stewed	1 (1.3 oz)	94	61	0

FOOD	PORTION	CAL	VIT A	VIT C
neck w/o skin, stewed	1 (.6 oz)	32	22	0
skin, batter dipped & fried	4 oz	449	158	0
skin, batter dipped & fried	from ½ chicken (6.7 oz)	748	263	0
skin, floured & fried	1 oz	166	77	0
skin, floured & fried	½ chicken (2 oz)	281	130	0
skin, roasted	½ chicken (2 oz)	254	146	0
skin, stewed	½ chicken (2.5 oz)	261	143	0
thigh w/ skin, batter dipped & fried	1 (3 oz)	238	82	0
thigh w/ skin, floured & fried	1 (2.2 oz)	162	61	0
thigh w/ skin, roasted	1 (2.2 oz)	153	102	0
thigh w/ skin, stewed	1 (2.4 oz)	158	103	0
thigh w/o skin, fried	1 (1.8 oz)	113	37	0
thigh w/o skin, roasted	1 (1.8 oz)	109	34	0
thigh w/o skin, stewed	1 (1.9 oz)	107	34	0
w/ skin, floured & fried	½ breast (3.4 oz)	218	49	0
w/ skin, floured fried	½ chicken (11 oz)	844	280	0
w/ skin, fried	½ chicken (16.4 oz)	1347	434	0
w/ skin, neck & giblets, batter dipped & fried	1 chicken (2.3 lbs)	2987	6202	4
w/ skin, neck & giblets, roasted	1 chicken (1.5 lbs)	1598	4340	4
w/ skin, neck & giblets, stewed	1 chicken (1.6 lbs)	1625	4350	4
w/ skin, roasted	½ chicken (10.5 oz)	715	482	0
w/ skin, stewed	½ chicken (11.7 oz)	730	488	0
w/o skin, roasted	1 cup (5 oz)	266	74	0
w/o skin, fried	1 cup	307	82	0
w/o skin, stewed	1 cup (5 oz)	248	70	0
w/o skin, stewed	1 oz	54	23	0
wing w/ skin, batter dipped & fried	1 (1.7 oz)	159	55	0
wing w/ skin, floured & fried	1 (1.1 oz)	103	40	0
wing w/ skin, roasted	1 (1.2 oz)	99	54	0
wing w/ skin, stewed	1 (1.4 oz)	100	53	0

FOOD	PORTION	CAL	VIT A	VIT C
capon w/ skin, neck & giblets, roasted	1 chicken (3.1 lbs)	3211	10408	6
roaster dark meat w/o skin, roasted	1 cup (5 oz)	250	76	0
roaster light meat w/o skin, roasted	1 cup (5 oz)	214	35	0
roaster w/ skin, neck & giblets, roasted	1 chicken (2.4 lbs)	2363	6400	4
roaster w/ skin, roasted	½ chicken (1.1 lbs)	1071	399	0
roaster w/o skin, roasted	1 cup (5 oz)	469	57	0
stewing dark meat w/o skin, stewed	1 cup (5 oz)	361	203	0
stewing w/ skin neck & giblets, stewed	1 chicken (1.3 lbs)	1636	5487	3
stewing w/ skin, stewed	½ chicken (9.2 oz)	744	343	0
stewing w/ skin, stewed	6.2 oz	507	234	0
FROZEN PREPARED Banquet Boneless Breast Tenders	2.25 oz	150	100	1
READY-TO-USE Carl Buddig	1 oz	60	0	0
poultry salad sandwich spread	1 oz	238	39	0
poultry salad sandwich spread	1 tbsp (13 g)	109	18	0
TAKE-OUT boneless breaded & fried w/ barbecue sauce	6 pieces (4.6 oz)	330	342	tr
breaded & fried w/ honey	6 pieces (4 oz)	339	101	tr
breaded & fried w/ mustard sauce	6 pieces (4.6 oz)	323	110	tr
breaded & fried w/ sweet & sour sauce	6 pieces (4.6 oz)	346	242	tr
breast & wing, breaded & fried	2 pieces (5.7 oz)	494	192	0

FOOD	PORTION	CAL	VIT A	VIT C
drumstick, breaded & fried	2 pieces (5.2 oz)	430	222	0
thigh, breaded & fried	2 pieces (5.2 oz)	430	222	0

CHICKEN DISHES

CANNED
Chicken Stew (Swanson)	7⅝ oz	160	5500	6

HOME RECIPE
chicken & noodles	1 cup	365	430	tr
chicken a la king	1 cup	470	1130	12

MIX
Lipton Microeasy Barbeque Chicken	¼ pkg	108	1614	17
Lipton Microeasy Country Chicken	¼ pkg	78	3125	58

TAKE-OUT
chicken cacciatore	¾ cup	394	1586	40
chicken & dumplings	¾ cup	256	233	4
chicken pie w/ top crust	1 slice (5.6 oz)	472	800	0
fillet sandwich, plain	1	515	100	9
fillet sandwich w/ cheese, lettuce, mayonnaise & tomato	1	632	620	3

CHICKPEAS

CANNED
Goya Spanish Style	7.5 oz	150	460	2
Green Giant Garbanzo	½ cup	90	0	0
S&W Garbanzo Premium Large	½ cup	110	100	4
S&W Garbanzo Water Pack	½ cup	105	100	1
chickpeas	1 cup	285	58	9

DRIED
cooked	1 cup	269	44	2

FOOD	PORTION	CAL	VIT A	VIT C
CHICORY				
FRESH				
greens, raw, chopped	½ cup	21	3600	22
root, raw	1 (2.1 oz)	44	4	3
roots, raw, cut up	½ cup (1.6 oz)	33	3	2
witloof head, raw	1 (1.9 oz)	9	15	2
witloof, raw	½ cup (1.5 oz)	8	13	1

CHILI
(Vegetarian chili will contain more plant sources of vitamin A.)

FOOD	PORTION	CAL	VIT A	VIT C
CANNED				
Gebhardt Hot With Beans	1 cup	470	293	40
Gebhardt Plain	1 cup	530	39	11
Gebhardt With Beans	1 cup	495	86	40
Health Valley Mild Vegetarian With Beans	5 oz	160	750	2
Health Valley Mild Vegetarian With Beans No Salt Added	5 oz	160	750	2
Health Valley Mild Vegetarian With Lentils	5 oz	140	1050	12
Health Valley Mild Vegetarian With Lentils No Salt Added	5 oz	140	1050	12
Health Valley Spicy Vegetarian With Beans	5 oz	160	950	2
Healthy Choice Spicy w/ Beans & Ground Turkey	½ can (7.5 oz)	210	1250	15
Healthy Choice Turkey w/ Beans	½ can (7.5 oz)	200	1500	12
Hunt's Chili Beans	4 oz	100	10	3
Just Rite Hot With Beans	4 oz	195	13	4
Just Rite With Beans	4 oz	200	7	4
Just Rite Without Beans	4 oz	180	8	5
Manwich Chili Fixin's, as prep	8 oz	290	200	24

FOOD	PORTION	CAL	VIT A	VIT C
S&W Chili Makin's Original	½ cup	100	1750	9
S&W Chili Beans	½ cup	130	500	4
Wolf Brand Plain	7.5 oz	330	3500	5
chili w/ beans	1 cup	286	860	4
DRIED				
powder	1 tsp	8	908	2
FROZEN				
Swanson Homestyle Chili Con Carne	8¼ oz	270	1250	4
TAKE-OUT				
con carne w/ beans	8.9 oz	254	1663	2

CHINESE PRESERVING MELON

cooked	½ cup	11	0	9

CHIPS

FOOD	PORTION	CAL	VIT A	VIT C
CORN				
Health Valley	1 oz	160	97	2
Health Valley No Salt Added	1 oz	160	97	2
Health Valley With Cheddar Cheese	1 oz	160	114	2
POTATO				
Old Dutch Foods	1 oz	150	tr	6
Old Dutch Foods Augratin	1 oz	150	tr	5
Old Dutch Foods BBQ	1 oz	140	tr	6
Old Dutch Foods Dill Flavored	1 oz	150	tr	6
Old Dutch Foods Onion & Garlic	1 oz	150	tr	12
Old Dutch Foods Ripple	1 oz	150	tr	6
Old Dutch Foods Sour Cream & Onion	1 oz	150	tr	9
potato	1 oz	152	0	9
potato	1 pkg (8 oz)	1217	0	71

FOOD	PORTION	CAL	VIT A	VIT C
sticks	1 pkg (1 oz)	148	0	13
sticks	½ cup	94	0	9

CHITTERLINGS
pork, simmered	3 oz	258	0	0

CHIVES
freeze-dried	1 tbsp	1	137	1
fresh, chopped	1 tbsp	1	131	2
fresh, chopped	1 tsp	0	44	1

CHOCOLATE
BAKING				
baking	1 oz	145	10	0
CHIPS				
Baker's Big Milk Chocolate	¼ cup	239	77	1
MIX				
powder	2–3 heaping tsp	75	4	tr
powder, as prep w/ whole milk	9 oz	226	312	3
SYRUP				
chocolate	1 cup	653	89	1
chocolate	2 tbsp	82	11	tr
chocolate as prep w/ whole milk	9 oz	232	319	2

CHUTNEY
apple	1.2 oz	68	5	1
tomato	1.2 oz	54	105	3

CILANTO
fresh	¼ cup	1	111	tr

CINNAMON
ground	1 tsp	6	6	1

FOOD	PORTION	CAL	VIT A	VIT C

CLAMS
(The vitamin A in prepared clam products comes from animal and/or plant sources.)

CANNED				
American Original Foods Quahogs	4 oz	66	150	1
FROZEN				
Microwave Fried Clams (Mrs. Paul's)	2.5 oz	260	tr	tr
TAKE-OUT				
breaded & fried	¾ cup	451	122	0

CLOVES

ground	1 tsp	7	11	2

COCOA
(The vitamin A in prepared cocoa products comes from animal and/or plant sources.)

Nestle Hot Cocoa Mix With Marshmallows, as prep w/ 2% milk	6 oz	220	400	1
Nestle Hot Cocoa Mix With Marshmallows, as prep w/ skim milk	6 oz	190	400	1
Nestle Hot Cocoa Mix With Marshmallows, as prep w/ whole milk	6 oz	240	200	1
Nestle Hot Cocoa Mix, as prep w/ 2% milk	6 oz	210	400	1
Nestle Hot Cocoa Mix, as prep w/ skim milk	6 oz	180	400	1
Nestle Hot Cocoa Mix, as prep w/ whole milk	6 oz	230	200	1
Ultra Slim-Fast Hot Cocoa, as prep w/ water	8 oz	190	1750	21
hot cocoa	1 cup	218	318	2
mix, as prep w/ water	7 oz	103	4	1

FOOD	PORTION	CAL	VIT A	VIT C
powder	1 oz	102	4	1

COCONUT

coconut water	1 cup	46	0	6
coconut water	1 tbsp	3	0	tr
dried, sweetened, flaked	1 cup	351	0	0
dried, sweetened, flaked	7 oz pkg	944	0	0
dried, sweetened, shredded	1 cup	466	0	1
dried, sweetened, shredded	7 oz pkg	997	0	1
dried, unsweetened	1 oz	187	0	tr
fresh	1 piece (1.5 oz)	159	0	2
fresh, shredded	1 cup	283	0	3

COD
(The vitamin A in cod is from animal sources.)

CANNED				
atlantic	1 can (11 oz)	327	144	1
atlantic	3 oz	89	39	1
DRIED				
atlantic	3 oz	246	120	3
FRESH				
atlantic, raw	3 oz	70	34	1
atlantic, cooked	1 fillet (6.3 oz)	189	83	2
atlantic, cooked	3 oz	89	39	1

COFFEE
(The vitamin A in coffee substitutes comes from animal sources.)

INSTANT				
cappuccino mix, as prep	7 oz	62	0	0
decaffeinated	1 rounded tsp	4	0	0
decaffeinated, as prep	6 oz	4	0	0

FOOD	PORTION	CAL	VIT A	VIT C
mocha mix, as prep	7 oz	51	0	0
regular	1 rounded tsp	4	0	0
regular, as prep	6 oz	4	0	0

COFFEE SUBSTITUTES

powder, as prep w/ milk	6 oz	121	230	2

COFFEE WHITENERS

LIQUID

nondairy, frzn	1 tbsp	20	13	0

POWDER

nondairy	1 tsp	11	4	0

COLLARDS

FRESH

cooked	½ cup	17	1745	8
raw, chopped	½ cup	6	599	4

FROZEN

chopped, cooked	½ cup	31	5084	23

COOKIES
(The vitamin A in cookies comes from non-plant ingredients like milk and eggs; the exception is fruit cookies, with some of the vitamin A coming from plant sources.)

HOME RECIPE

chocolate chip	4 (1.5 oz)	185	20	0
peanut butter	4 (1.7 oz)	245	20	0
shortbread	2 (1 oz)	145	300	tr

READY-TO-EAT

Amaranth Cookies (Health Valley)	1	70	88	3
Chocolate Chip (Drake's)	2 (1 oz)	140	tr	tr
Chocolate-Chocolate Chip (Drake's)	2 (1 oz)	130	tr	tr

FOOD	PORTION	CAL	VIT A	VIT C
Coconut (Drake's)	2 (1 oz)	130	tr	tr
Coconut Macaroon (Drake's)	1 (1 oz)	135	tr	tr
Fancy Fruit Chunks (Health Valley)				
Apricot Almond	2	90	217	3
Date Pecan	2	90	6	3
Raisin Oat Bran	2	70	4	2
Tropical Fruit	2	90	216	3
Fancy Peanut Chunks (Health Valley)	2	90	4	3
Fat Free Hawaiian Fruit (Health Valley)	3	75	200	4
Fat Free Apricot Delight (Health Valley)	3	75	300	4
Fortune (La Choy)	1	15	tr	0
Fruit & Fitness (Health Valley)	5	200	1257	3
Fruit Jumbos Almond Date (Health Valley)	1	70	1	3
Fruit Jumbos Raisin Nut (Health Valley)	1	70	1	3
Fruit Jumbos Tropical Fruit (Health Valley)	1	70	513	3
Fruit Jumbos Oat Bran (Health Valley)	1	70	8	tr
Graham Amaranth (Health Valley)	7	110	0	5
Graham Honey (Health Valley)	7	100	1	4
Graham Oat Bran (Health Valley)	7	120	1	4
Hermit (Drake's)	1 (2 oz)	230	tr	tr
Honey Jumbos Crisp Cinnamon (Health Valley)	1	70	3	3
Honey Jumbos Crisp Peanut Butter (Health Valley)	1	70	tr	2

FOOD	PORTION	CAL	VIT A	VIT C
Honey Jumbos Fancy Oat Bran (Health Valley)	2	130	1	tr
Oat Bran Animal Cookies (Health Valley)	7	110	2	3
Oat Bran Fruit & Nut (Health Valley)	2	110	3	3
Oatmeal (Drake's)	2 (1 oz)	120	tr	tr
Oatmeal Creme (Drake's)	1 (2 oz)	240	tr	tr
Peanut Butter Wafers (Drake's)	1 (2.25 oz)	324	tr	tr
The Great Tofu (Health Valley)	2	90	99	3
The Great Wheat Free (Health Valley)	2	80	3	4
animal crackers	1 box (2.4 oz)	299	27	tr
chocolate sandwich	4 (1.4 oz)	195	0	0
chocolate chip	1 box (1.9 oz)	233	52	tr
chocolate chip	4 (1.5 oz)	180	50	tr
digestive biscuits, plain	2	141	0	0
fig bars	4 (2 oz)	210	60	tr
graham	2 squares	60	0	0
oatmeal raisin	4 (1.8 oz)	245	40	0
shortbread	4 (1 oz)	155	30	0
vanilla sandwich	4 (1.4 oz)	195	0	0
vanilla wafers	10 (1.25 oz)	185	50	0
REFRIGERATED				
Chocolate Chip	1	70	0	0
Oatmeal Raisin (Pillsbury)	1	60	0	0
Peanut Butter (Pillsbury)	1	70	0	0
Sugar (Pillsbury)	1	70	0	0
chocolate chip	4 (1.7 oz)	225	30	0
sugar	4 (1.7 oz)	235	40	0

FOOD	PORTION	CAL	VIT A	VIT C

CORN

CANNED

FOOD	PORTION	CAL	VIT A	VIT C
50% Less Salt No Sugar Added (Green Giant)	½ cup	50	100	0
Corn (Green Giant)	½ cup	70	100	4
Cream Style (Green Giant)	½ cup	100	100	2
Cream Style Premium Homestyle (S&W)	½ cup	105	100	2
Cream Style Diet (S&W)	½ cup	100	500	7
Deli Corn (Green Giant)	½ cup	80	300	0
Golden Kernel 50% Less Salt (Green Giant)	½ cup	70	0	2
Golden Vacuum Packed (Green Giant)	½ cup	80	200	6
Mexi Corn (Green Giant)	½ cup	80	200	4
No Salt No Sugar (Green Giant)	½ cup	80	100	2
Sweet 'N Natural (S&W)	½ cup	90	400	5
Sweet Select (Green Giant)	½ cup	60	100	0
White Vacuum Packed (Green Giant)	½ cup	80	0	6
Whole Kernel Tender Young (S&W)	½ cup	90	200	5
Whole Kernel Water Pack (S&W)	½ cup	80	500	5
cream style	½ cup	93	124	6
w/ red & green peppers	½ cup	86	265	10
FRESH				
on-the-cob, cooked, w/ butter	1 ear	155	391	7
white, cooked	½ cup	89	tr	5
white, raw	½ cup	66	tr	5
yellow, cooked	1 ear (2.7 oz)	83	167	5
yellow, cooked	½ cup	89	178	5

FOOD	PORTION	CAL	VIT A	VIT C
yellow, raw	1 ear (3 oz)	77	253	6
yellow raw	½ cup	66	216	5
FROZEN				
Big Ears (Birds Eye)	1 ear	160	300	9
Cob Corn (Ore Ida)	1 ear (5.3 oz)	190	400	12
Cob Corn Mini-Gold (Ore Ida)	1 (2.65 oz)	90	200	5
Cream Style (Green Giant)	½ cup	110	100	5
Cut (Big Valley)	3.5 oz	80	200	5
Harvest Fresh Niblets (Green Giant)	½ cup	80	0	4
Harvest Fresh White Shoepeg (Green Giant)	½ cup	90	0	6
In Butter Sauce (Birds Eye)	½ cup	90	200	4
In Butter Sauce (Green Giant)	½ cup	100	0	2
Little Ears (Birds Eye)	2 ears	130	300	9
Nibblers Corn On The Cob (Green Giant)	2 ears	120	100	5
Niblet Ears (Green Giant)	1 ear	120	100	5
Niblets (Green Giant)	½ cup	90	0	4
On The Cob (Birds Eye)	1 ear	120	300	9
One Serve Niblets In Butter Sauce (Green Giant)	1 pkg	120	100	5
One Serve On The Cob (Green Giant)	1 pkg	120	100	0
Polybag Cut (Birds Eye)	½ cup	80	200	5
Polybag Deluxe Tender Sweet (Birds Eye)	½ cup	80	200	5
Super Sweet Nibblers Corn On The Cob (Green Giant)	2 ears	90	200	2
Super Sweet Niblet Ears (Green Giant)	1 ear	90	200	2
Super Sweet Niblet Select (Green Giant)	½ cup	60	100	0

FOOD	PORTION	CAL	VIT A	VIT C
Sweet (Birds Eye)	½ cup	80	200	5
White Select (Green Giant)	½ cup	90	0	6
White In Butter Sauce (Green Giant)	½ cup	100	0	5
cooked	½ cup	67	204	2
on-the-cob, cooked	1 ear (2.2 oz)	59	133	3
SHELF STABLE Golden Whole Kernel (Pantry Express)	½ cup	60	300	1
TAKE-OUT fritters	1 (1 oz)	62	66	1
scalloped	½ cup	258	620	14
CORNMEAL				
Aunt Jemima White	3 tbsp	102	0	0
Aunt Jemima Yellow	3 tbsp	102	115	0
Quaker White	3 tbsp	102	0	0
Quaker Yellow	3 tbsp	102	115	0
degermed	1 cup	506	570	0
whole grain	1 cup	442	573	0
HOME RECIPE hush puppies	1 (¾ oz)	74	31	0
hush puppies	5 (2.7 oz)	256	94	0
MIX Aunt Jemima Bolted White Mix	3 tbsp	99	0	0
Aunt Jemima Buttermilk Self-Rising White Mix	3 tbsp	101	0	0
Aunt Jemima Self Rising Yellow Mix	3 tbsp	100	0	0
Aunt Jemima Self-Rising White Mix	3 tbsp	98	0	0

FOOD	PORTION	CAL	VIT A	VIT C

COTTAGE CHEESE
(The vitamin A in cottage cheese comes from animal sources.)

FOOD	PORTION	CAL	VIT A	VIT C
creamed	1 cup	217	342	tr
creamed	4 oz	117	184	tr
creamed w/ fruit	4 oz	140	139	tr
dry curd	1 cup	123	44	0
dry curd	4 oz	96	34	0
lowfat 1%	1 cup	164	84	tr
lowfat 1%	4 oz	82	42	tr
lowfat 2%	1 cup	203	158	tr
lowfat 2%	4 oz	101	79	tr

COWPEAS

FOOD	PORTION	CAL	VIT A	VIT C
CANNED				
common	1 cup	184	32	7
DRIED				
catjang, cooked	1 cup	200	17	1
FRESH				
leafy tips, chopped, cooked	1 cup	12	305	10
leafy tips, raw, chopped	1 cup	10	256	13
FROZEN				
cooked	½ cup	112	64	2

CRAB

FOOD	PORTION	CAL	VIT A	VIT C
TAKE-OUT				
baked	1 (3.8 oz)	160	78	3
cake	1 (2 oz)	160	313	tr
soft-shell fried	1 (4.4 oz)	334	15	tr

CRACKER CRUMBS

FOOD	PORTION	CAL	VIT A	VIT C
Corn Flake Crumbs (Kellogg's)	¼ cup (1 oz)	100	0	15

FOOD	PORTION	CAL	VIT A	VIT C
CRACKERS				
Butter Crackers (Goya)	1	40	<100	0
Goya Crackers	1	30	<100	0
Herb Stoned Wheat No Salt (Health Valley)	13	55	50	1
Rice Bran (Health Valley)	7	130	15	2
Sesame Stoned Wheat (Health Valley)	13	55	50	1
Stoned Wheat (Health Valley)	13	55	50	1
cheese	10 (1.3 oz)	50	20	0
crispbread	3	61	0	0
crispbread, rye	3	77	0	0
melba toast, plain	1	20	0	0
peanut butter sandwich	1 (⅓ oz)	40	tr	0
saltines	4	50	0	0
water biscuits	3	92	0	0
CRANBERRIES				
CANNED				
cranberry sauce, sweetened	½ cup	209	28	3
FRESH				
chopped	1 cup	54	50	15
JUICE				
cranberry juice cocktail	6 oz	108	7	67
cranberry juice cocktail, frzn	12 oz can	821	148	148
cranberry juice cocktail, frzn, as prep	6 oz	102	18	18
CRANBERRY BEANS				
CANNED				
cranberry beans	1 cup	216	0	2
DRIED				
cooked	1 cup	240	0	0

FOOD	PORTION	CAL	VIT A	VIT C

CREAM
(The vitamin A in cream comes from animal sources.)

LIQUID

FOOD	PORTION	CAL	VIT A	VIT C
half & half	1 cup	315	1050	2
half & half	1 tbsp	20	65	tr
heavy whipping	1 tbsp	52	220	tr
light coffee	1 cup	496	1728	2
light coffee	1 tbsp	29	108	tr
light whipping	1 tbsp	44	169	tr
WHIPPED				
heavy whipping	1 cup	411	3499	1
light whipping	1 cup	345	2694	1

CREAM CHEESE
(The vitamin A cream cheese comes from animal sources.)

FOOD	PORTION	CAL	VIT A	VIT C
NEUFCHATEL				
neufchatel	1 oz	74	321	0
neufchatel	1 pkg (3 oz)	221	964	0
REDUCED CALORIE				
Fleur De Lait Alouette C'est Light Strawberry	1 oz	75	200	4
Fleur De Lait Ultra Light Strawberry	1 oz	70	100	1
REGULAR				
cream cheese	1 oz	99	405	0
cream cheese	1 pkg (3 oz)	297	1213	0

CREAM OF TARTAR

FOOD	PORTION	CAL	VIT A	VIT C
cream of tartar	1 tsp	8	0	0

CRESS

FOOD	PORTION	CAL	VIT A	VIT C
garden, cooked	½ cup	16	5236	16
garden, raw	½ cup	8	2325	17

FOOD	PORTION	CAL	VIT A	VIT C

CROISSANT
(The vitamin A in croissants comes from animal ingredients like butter and eggs.)

FOOD	PORTION	CAL	VIT A	VIT C
croissant	1 (2 oz)	235	50	0
TAKE-OUT				
w/ egg & cheese	1	369	1000	tr
w/ egg, cheese & bacon	1	413	472	2
w/ egg, cheese & ham	1	475	451	11
w/ egg, cheese & sausage	1	524	422	tr

CROUTONS

Kellogg's Croutettes	1 cup (1 oz)	100	0	tr

CUCUMBER

FRESH				
raw	1 (11 oz)	38	647	16
raw, sliced	½ cup (1.8 oz)	7	112	3
TAKE-OUT				
cucumber salad	3.5 oz	50	750	9

CUMIN

seed	1 tsp	8	27	tr

CURRANTS

DRIED				
zante	½ cup	204	52	3
FRESH				
black	½ cup	36	129	101
JUICE				
black currant nectar	3 ½ oz	55	tr	30
red currant nectar	3 ½ oz	54	tr	6

FOOD	PORTION	CAL	VIT A	VIT C

CUSTARD
(the vitamin A in custard comes from non-plant sources.)

FOOD	PORTION	CAL	VIT A	VIT C
Flan (Jell-O)	½ cup	151	154	1
Golden Egg Americana (Jell-O)	½ cup	160	230	1
baked	1 cup	305	530	1
zabaglione, home recipe	½ cup	135	485	0

DANDELION GREENS

FOOD	PORTION	CAL	VIT A	VIT C
fresh, cooked	½ cup	17	6084	9
raw, chopped	½ cup	13	3920	10

DANISH PASTRY
(The vitamin A in danish pastry comes from animal ingredients like eggs and milk; the exception is fruit danish, with some of the vitamin A coming from plant sources.)

FOOD	PORTION	CAL	VIT A	VIT C
READY-TO-EAT				
cheese	1 (3 oz)	353	155	3
cinnamon	1 (3 oz)	349	18	3
fruit	1 (2.3 oz)	235	40	tr
fruit	1 (3.3 oz)	335	86	2
plain	1 (2 oz)	220	60	tr
plain ring	1 (12 oz)	1305	360	tr
REFRIGERATED				
Caramel Danish w/ Nuts (Pillsbury)	1	160	0	0
Cinnamon Raisin Danish w/ Icing (Pillsbury)	1	150	0	0
Orange Danish w/ Icing (Pillsbury)	1	150	0	0

DATES

FOOD	PORTION	CAL	VIT A	VIT C
DRIED				
Bordo Diced	2 oz	203	tr	12
Dole Chopped	½ cup	280	9	8

FOOD	PORTION	CAL	VIT A	VIT C
chopped	1 cup	489	89	0
whole	10	228	42	0

DINNER
(The vitamin A in dinners comes from both animal and plant sources.)

FROZEN
Armour Classics

Chicken Fettucini	11 oz	260	1500	60
Chicken Parmigiana	11.5 oz	370	750	9
Chicken & Noodles	11 oz	230	4500	54
Chicken Mesquite	9.5 oz	370	400	15
Chicken w/ Wine & Mushroom Sauce	10.75 oz	280	1750	21
Glazed Chicken	10.75 oz	300	300	9
Meat Loaf	11.25 oz	360	300	9
Salisbury Parmigiana	11.5 oz	410	300	6
Salisbury Steak	11.25 oz	350	300	24
Swedish Meatballs	11.25 oz	330	2500	9
Turkey w/ Dressing & Gravy	11.5 oz	320	3000	6
Veal Parmigiana	11.25 oz	400	1000	27

Armour Lite

Beef Pepper Steak	11.25 oz	220	500	15
Beef Stroganoff	11.25 oz	250	2500	42
Chicken Marsala	10.5 oz	250	300	18
Chicken Ala King	11.25 oz	290	2250	60
Chicken Burgundy	10 oz	210	2000	24
Chicken Oriental	10 oz	180	500	42
Salisbury Steak	11.5 oz	300	300	12
Shrimp Creole	11.25 oz	260	300	14
Sweet & Sour Chicken	11 oz	240	1000	24

FOOD	PORTION	CAL	VIT A	VIT C
Banquet				
Boneless Chicken Drumsnacker Platter	7 oz	290	100	6
Extra Helping Beef Dinner	15.5 oz	430	2000	9
Extra Helping Turkey Dinner	17 oz	460	200	1
Birds Eye				
Easy Recipe Beef Burgundy, not prep	½ pkg	120	1500	9
Easy Recipe Beef Fajitas, not prep	½ pkg	80	2250	60
Budget Gourmet				
Beef Cantonese	1 pkg	260	3000	24
Beef Stroganoff	1 pkg	290	750	9
Breast of Chicken In Wine Sauce	1 pkg	250	2250	24
Chicken Cacciatore	1 pkg	470	1500	36
Chicken And Egg Noodle w/ Broccoli	1 pkg	440	1000	12
Chicken Au Gratin	1 pkg	250	1250	12
Chicken Marsala	1 pkg	270	1750	5
Chicken With Fettucini	1 pkg	400	1250	4
French Recipe Chicken	1 pkg	240	3000	6
Glazed Turkey	1 pkg	270	100	2
Ham & Asparagus Au Gratin	1 pkg	290	100	5
Light And Healthy Chicken Breast Parmigiana	1 pkg	260	5000	27
Light And Healthy Herbed Chicken Breast With Fettucini	1 pkg	240	3000	24
Light And Healthy Italian Style Meatloaf	1 pkg	270	5000	36
Light And Healthy Pot Roast	1 pkg	210	5000	9

FOOD	PORTION	CAL	VIT A	VIT C
Budget Gourmet *(cont.)*				
Light And Healthy Sirloin Beef In Wine Sauce	1 pkg	230	4500	9
Light And Healthy Sirloin Salisbury Steak	1 pkg	260	3250	18
Light And Healthy Special Recipe Sirloin Of Beef	1 pkg	250	5000	6
Light And Healthy Stuffed Turkey Breast	1 pkg	230	3000	60
Light and Healthy Teriyaki Chicken Breast	1 pkg	310	1250	36
Mandarin Chicken	1 pkg	300	1500	15
Orange Glazed Chicken	1 pkg	250	750	12
Oriental Beef	1 pkg	290	1500	18
Pepper Steak With Rice	1 pkg	330	1000	15
Roast Chicken With Herb Gravy	1 pkg	270	1500	15
Roast Sirloin Supreme	1 pkg	320	200	5
Scallops and Shrimp Marinara	1 pkg	330	1250	36
Seafood Newburg	1 pkg	350	400	2
Sirloin Beef In Herb Sauce	1 pkg	270	1000	5
Sirloin Cheddar Melt	1 pkg	390	500	12
Sirloin Salisbury Steak	1 pkg	260	5000	4
Sirloin Salisbury Steak Dinner	1 pkg	450	1250	27
Sirloin Tips In Burgundy Sauce	1 pkg	340	2000	12
Sirloin Tips With Country Vegetables	1 pkg	300	2500	15
Sliced Turkey Breast With Herb Gravy	1 pkg	290	5000	15
Swedish Meatballs With Noodles	1 pkg	580	750	2

FOOD	PORTION	CAL	VIT A	VIT C
Sweet & Sour Chicken	1 pkg	340	2000	9
Swiss Steak With Zesty Tomato Sauce	1 pkg	410	4500	12
Turkey A La King With Rice	1 pkg	390	750	2
Veal Parmigiana	1 pkg	490	10000	15
Yankee Pot Roast	1 pkg	360	2500	9
Dining Light Salisbury Steak	9 oz	200	500	2
Healthy Choice				
Barbecue Beef Ribs	11 oz	330	300	5
Beef Pepper Steak	11 oz	290	400	72
Breast of Turkey	10.5 oz	290	200	48
Cacciatore Chicken	12.5 oz	310	500	6
Chicken Parmigiana	11.5 oz	270	4500	26
Chicken & Pasta Divan	11.5 oz	310	3500	72
Chicken A L'Orange	9 oz	240	750	27
Chicken And Vegetables	11.5 oz	210	750	9
Chicken Dijon	11 oz	260	750	30
Chicken Oriental	11.25 oz	230	300	30
Herb Roasted Chicken	12.3 oz	290	750	38
Lemon Pepper Fish	10.7 oz	300	400	48
Mandarin Chicken	11 oz	260	1250	9
Mesquite Chicken	10.5 oz	340	750	138
Salisbury Steak	11.5 oz	300	100	72
Salsa Chicken	11.25 oz	240	1000	60
Shrimp Creole	11.25 oz	230	400	84
Shrimp Marinara	10.25 oz	260	500	114
Sirloin Beef With Barbecue Sauce	11 oz	300	750	27
Sirloin Tips	11.75 oz	280	3500	42
Sole Au Gratin	11 oz	270	100	6
Sweet & Sour Chicken	11.5 oz	280	300	84

FOOD	PORTION	CAL	VIT A	VIT C
Healthy Choice *(cont.)*				
Turkey Tetrazzini	12.6 oz	340	100	72
Yankee Pot Roast	11 oz	250	500	9
Kid Cuisine				
Chicken Sandwiches	8.2 oz	470	300	2
Mexican Style	5.7 oz	290	100	6
Le Menu				
Beef Sirloin Tips	11½ oz	400	300	15
Beef Stroganoff	10 oz	430	500	1
Chicken Parmigiana	11¾ oz	410	400	6
Chicken A La King	10¼ oz	330	300	4
Chicken Corden Bleu	11 oz	460	7000	4
Chicken In Wine Sauce	10 oz	280	4000	4
Chopped Sirloin Beef	12¼ oz	430	100	5
Ham Steak	10 oz	300	6000	18
LightStyle Herb Roasted Chicken	10 oz	240	400	18
LightStyle Sliced Turkey	10 oz	210	3500	36
LightStyle Sweet And Sour Chicken	10 oz	250	2000	36
LightStyle Turkey Divan	10 oz	260	750	36
Pepper Steak	11½ oz	370	1000	6
Sliced Breast of Turkey With Mushroom Gravy	10½ oz	300	2500	9
Sweet & Sour Chicken	11¼ oz	400	1000	4
Veal Parmigiana	11½ oz	390	750	6
Yankee Pot Roast	10 oz	330	6000	6
Le Menu Entree				
LightStyle Chicken Dijon	8 oz	240	1250	6
LightStyle Empress Chicken	8¼ oz	210	1500	9
LightStyle Glazed Turkey	8¼ oz	260	100	4
LightStyle Herb Roast Chicken	7¾ oz	260	350	1

FOOD	PORTION	CAL	VIT A	VIT C
LightStyle Traditional Turkey	8 oz	200	1500	12
Lean Cuisine				
Beefsteak Ranchero	9.25 oz	260	500	6
Breaded Breast of Chicken Parmesan	10.9 oz	270	1500	6
Breast of Chicken Marsala With Vegetables	8.1 oz	190	1500	9
Chicken Cacciatore With Vermicelli	10.9 oz	280	500	9
Chicken Tenderloins In Herb Cream Sauce	9½ oz	240	1000	5
Chicken Tenderloins In Peanut Sauce	9 oz	290	400	5
Chicken & Vegetables With Vermicelli	11.75 oz	250	750	6
Chicken A l'Orange With Almond Rice	8 oz	280	400	12
Chicken In Barbecue Sauce	8¾ oz	260	1250	18
Chicken Oriental With Vegetables And Vermicelli	9 oz	280	200	6
Fiesta Chicken	8½ oz	240	750	9
Filet of Fish Divan	10.4 oz	210	100	27
Filet of Fish Florentine	9.6 oz	220	2500	1
Glazed Chicken With Vegetable Rice	8.5 oz	260	100	4
Homestyle Turkey With Vegetables and Pasta	9⅜ oz	230	1500	1
Oriental Beef With Vegetables And Rice	8.6 oz	290	750	1
Sliced Turkey Breast In Mushroom Sauce	8 oz	220	750	2
Sliced Turkey Breast With Dressing	7⅞ oz	200	2500	6
Stuffed Cabbage With Meat In Tomato Sauce	10.75 oz	210	400	6

FOOD	PORTION	CAL	VIT A	VIT C
Lean Cuisine *(cont.)*				
Turkey Dijon	9.5 oz	230	2250	1
Morton				
Beans & Franks With Sauce	8.5 oz	300	4000	9
Glazed Ham	8 oz	230	2500	60
Gravy & Salisbury Steak	9 oz	270	3000	4
Veal Parmagian	8.75 oz	230	3000	2
Swanson				
Beans & Franks	10½ oz	440	300	9
Beef	11¼ oz	310	300	5
Beef in Barbecue Sauce	11 oz	460	1250	5
Chopped Sirloin Beef	10¾ oz	340	5000	4
Fish 'n' Chips	10 oz	500	400	2
Fried Chicken Dark Meat	9¾ oz	560	100	4
Fried Chicken White Meat	10¼ oz	550	100	2
Homestyle Chicken Cacciatore	10.95 oz	260	750	21
Homestyle Scalloped Potatoes And Ham	9 oz	300	200	9
Homestyle Seafood Creole With Rice	9 oz	240	750	30
Homestyle Sirloin Tips In Burgundy Sauce	7 oz	160	4000	27
Homestyle Turkey With Dressing & Potatoes	9 oz	290	300	2
Homestyle Veal Parmigiana	10 oz	330	300	6
Hungry-Man Boneless Chicken	17¾ oz	700	500	6
Hungry-Man Chopped Beef Steak	16¾ oz	640	400	9
Hungry-Man Salisbury Steak	16½ oz	680	400	6
Hungry-Man Sliced Beef	15¼ oz	450	500	6

FOOD	PORTION	CAL	VIT A	VIT C
Hungry-Man Turkey	17 oz	550	400	9
Hungry-Man Veal Parmigiana	18¼ oz	590	1000	15
Loin of Pork	10¾ oz	280	5000	6
Macaroni & Beef	12 oz	370	400	12
Meatloaf	10¾ oz	360	750	9
Noodles & Chicken	10½ oz	280	4000	2
Salisbury Steak	10¾ oz	400	200	4
Swiss Steak	10 oz	350	300	9
Turkey	11½ oz	350	300	5
Veal Parmigiana	12¼ oz	430	500	6
Western Style	11½ oz	430	500	12
Ultra Slim-Fast				
Beef Pepper Steak	12 oz	270	400	30
Chicken & Vegetable	12 oz	290	2000	2
Country Style Vegetable & Beef Tips	12 oz	230	4000	5
Mesquite Chicken	12 oz	360	1000	15
Roasted Chicken In Mushroom Sauce	12 oz	280	1750	1
Shrimp Creole	12 oz	240	750	27
Shrimp Marinara	12 oz	290	750	12
Sweet & Sour Chicken	12 oz	330	250	24

DIP
(The vitamin A in dip comes from animal sources.)

Nacho Cheese Premium (Kraft)	2 tbsp	55	100	1

DOCK

fresh, cooked	3½ oz	20	3474	26
raw, chopped	½ cup	15	2680	32

FOOD	PORTION	CAL	VIT A	VIT C

DOUGHNUTS

FOOD	PORTION	CAL	VIT A	VIT C
Old Fashion Donuts (Drake's)	1 (1.7 oz)	182	tr	tr
Powdered Sugar Donut Delites (Drake's)	7 (2.5 oz)	300	tr	tr
cake type	1 (1.8 oz)	210	20	tr
glazed	1 (2 oz)	235	tr	0

DRINK MIXER

FOOD	PORTION	CAL	VIT A	VIT C
whiskey sour mix	2 oz	55	14	2

DUCK
(The vitamin A in duck comes from animal source.)

FRESH

FOOD	PORTION	CAL	VIT A	VIT C
w/ skin, roasted	½ duck (13.4 oz)	1287	804	0
w/ skin, roasted	6 oz	583	364	0
w/o skin, roasted	½ duck (7.8 oz)	445	171	0
w/o skin, roasted	3.5 oz	201	77	0
wild, breast w/o skin, raw	½ breast (2.9 oz)	102	44	5

DURIAN

FOOD	PORTION	CAL	VIT A	VIT C
fresh	3½ oz	141	tr	42

EGG
(The vitamin A in eggs comes from the yolk, an animal source.)

CHICKEN

FOOD	PORTION	CAL	VIT A	VIT C
fried w/ margarine	1	91	394	0
frozen	1	75	317	0
frozen	1 cup	363	1543	0
hard cooked	1	77	280	0
hard cooked, chopped	1 cup	210	762	0
poached	1	74	316	0

FOOD	PORTION	CAL	VIT A	VIT C
raw	1	75	317	0
scrambled, plain	2	200	835	3
scrambled w/ whole milk & margarine	1	101	416	0
scrambled w/ whole milk & margarine	1 cup	365	1500	1
OTHER POULTRY duck, raw	1	130	930	0
quail, raw	1	14	27	0

EGG DISHES

FROZEN Great Starts Omelets With Cheese And Ham	7 oz	390	750	1
Quaker Scrambled Eggs, Cheddar Cheese & Fried Potatoes	1 pkg (5.9 oz)	250	300	9
Quaker Scrambled Eggs & Sausage With Hash Browns	1 pkg (5.7 oz)	290	300	4
HOME RECIPE deviled	2 halves	145	285	0
TAKE-OUT salad	½ cup	307	578	0
sandwich w/ cheese	1	340	668	2
sandwich w/ cheese & ham	1	348	561	3

EGG SUBSTITUTES

liquid	1½ oz	40	1015	0
liquid	1 cup	211	5422	0
powder	0.35 oz	44	122	tr
powder	0.7 oz	88	243	tr

EGGNOG
(The vitamin A in eggnog comes from animal sources.)

eggnog	1 cup	342	894	4

FOOD	PORTION	CAL	VIT A	VIT C
eggnog	1 qt	1368	3576	15
eggnog flavor mix, as prep w/ milk	9 oz	260	307	2

EGGPLANT
FRESH

cubed, cooked	½ cup	13	31	1
raw, cut up	½ cup (1.4 oz)	11	35	1
whole, peeled, raw	1 (1 lb)	117	387	8

ELDERBERRIES

fresh	1 cup	105	870	52

ENDIVE

raw, chopped	½ cup	4	513	2

ENGLISH MUFFIN
(The vitamin A comes from animal sources such as eggs and cheese.)

FROZEN

Healthy Choice English Muffin Sandwich	1 (4.5 oz)	200	300	4
Healthy Choice Western Style Omelet on English Muffin	1 (4.75 oz)	200	500	4

READY-TO-EAT

Thomas'	1	130	26	tr
Thomas' Honey Wheat	1	128	37	tr
Thomas' Raisin Cinnamon	1	151	52	tr
Thomas' Sour Dough	1	131	40	tr
whole wheat	1	134	0	0

TAKE-OUT

w/ butter	1	189	136	tr
w/ cheese & sausage	1	394	379	1

FOOD	PORTION	CAL	VIT A	VIT C
w/ egg, cheese & bacon	1	487	660	1
w/ egg, cheese & canadian bacon	1	383	594	1

EPPAW
raw	½ cup	75	0	7

FALAFEL
falafel	3 (1.8 oz)	170	7	1

FAT
Wesson shortening	1 tbcp	100	0	0
beef, cooked	1 oz	193	0	0
pork, cooked	1 oz	200	4	0

FEIJOA
fresh	1 (1.75 oz)	25	0	7
puree	1 cup	119	0	32

FIGS
CANNED				
in heavy syrup	3	75	31	1
in light syrup	3	58	32	1
water pack	3	42	31	1
DRIED				
cooked	1/2 cup	140	207	6
whole	10	477	248	2
FRESH				
fig	1 med	50	71	1

FILBERTS
dried, unblanched	1 oz	179	19	tr

FOOD	PORTION	CAL	VIT A	VIT C

FISH
(The vitamin A in fish comes from animal sources.)

FROZEN
Mrs. Paul's

40 Crunchy Fish Sticks	4 (2.75 oz)	200	tr	tr
Combination Seafood Platter	9 oz	600	tr	tr
Light Seafood Entrees Fish Florentine	8 oz	220	100	5
Light Seafood Entrees Fish Mornay	9 oz	230	100	21
Microwave Buttered Fillet	1 fillet	80	tr	12
Microwave Fillet Sandwich	1	280	tr	tr
Microwave Fillets	1 fillet	280	tr	tr
Microwave Fish Sticks	5	290	tr	tr
TAKE-OUT				
kedgeree	5.6 oz	242	640	0
sandwich w/ tartar sauce	1	431	110	3
sandwich w/ tartar sauce & cheese	1	524	432	3

FLATFISH

battered & fried	3.2 oz	211	35	0
breaded & fried	3.2 oz	211	35	0

FLOUR

All Purpose (Ballard)	1 cup	400	0	0
All Purpose Best (Pillsbury)	1 cup	400	0	0
Bohemian Style Rye and Wheat Best (Pillsbury)	1 cup	400	0	0
Bread Best (Pillsbury)	1 cup	400	0	0
Rye Medium Best (Pillsbury)	1 cup	400	0	0
Self-Rising (Aunt Jemima)	¼ cup	109	0	0

FOOD	PORTION	CAL	VIT A	VIT C
Self-Rising (Ballard)	1 cup	380	0	0
Self-Rising Best (Pillsbury)	1 cup	380	0	0
Shake & Blend Best (Pillsbury)	2 tbsp	50	0	0
Unbleached Best (Pillsbury)	1 cup	400	0	0
Whole Wheat Best (Pillsbury)	1 cup	400	0	0
cottonseed, lowfat	1 oz	94	123	1
peanut, defatted	1 cup	196	0	0
peanut, defatted	1 oz	92	0	0
potato	1 cup (6.3 oz)	628	0	34

FRENCH BEANS

dried, cooked	1 cup	228	5	2

FRENCH TOAST
(The vitamin A in French toast comes from animal ingredients such as eggs, milk and butter.)

FROZEN				
Aunt Jemima	3 oz	166	145	tr
Aunt Jemima Cinnamon Swirl	3 oz	171	163	tr
HOME RECIPE				
as prep w/ 2% milk	1 slice	149	315	tr
as prep w/ whole milk	1 slice	151	298	tr
TAKE-OUT				
w/ butter	2 slices	356	472	tr

FROG'S LEGS

frog leg, as prep w/ seasoned flour & fried	1 (0.8 oz)	70	0	0

FRUIT DRINKS

FROZEN				
Tree Top Apple Citrus, as prep	6 oz	90	60	15

FOOD	PORTION	CAL	VIT A	VIT C
citrus juice drink, as prep	1 cup	114	103	67
citrus juice drink, not prep	1 can (12 fl oz)	684	618	403
fruit punch, not prep	1 can (12 fl oz)	678	161	650
fruit punch, as prep w/ water	1 cup	113	27	108
lemonade	1 can (6 oz)	397	209	39
lemonade, as prep w/ water	1 cup	100	53	10
MIX				
fruit punch, as prep w/ water	9 oz	97	1	31
lemonade powder w/ Nutrasweet	1 pitcher (67 oz)	40	0	47
lemonade powder, as prep w/ water	9 oz	113	0	34
READY-TO-DRINK				
Dole New Breakfast Juice Pineapple Orange Banana	6 fl oz	90	200	60
Dole New Breakfast Juice Pineapple Orange Guava	6 fl oz	100	200	60
Dole New Breakfast Juice Pineapple Passion Banana	6 fl oz	100	200	60
Dole Pineapple Orange	6 fl oz	90	100	60
Dole Pineapple Orange Banana	6 fl oz	90	200	60
Kern's Apricot Orange Nectar	6 fl oz	112	1750	27
Kern's Apricot Pineapple Nectar	6 fl oz	110	1500	24
Kool-Aid Koolers Mountainberry Punch	1 pkg (8.45 fl oz)	142	1	6
Kool-Aid Koolers Rainbow Punch	1 pkg (8.45 fl oz)	135	1	6
Kool-Aid Koolers Sharkleberry Fin	1 pkg (8.45 fl oz)	140	1	6
Kool-Aid Koolers Tropical Punch	1 pkg (8.45 fl oz)	132	5	6
S&W Apricot Pineapple Nectar	6 fl oz	120	2000	1

FOOD	PORTION	CAL	VIT A	VIT C
S&W Apricot Pineapple Nectar Diet	6 fl oz	80	2500	30
Smucker's Orange Banana Juice	8 oz	120	100	36
Tang Mixed Fruit	8.45 fl oz	137	6	60
Tang Strawberry	8.45 fl oz	121	2	60
Tang Tropical Orange	8.45 fl oz	146	6	60
Tree Top Apple Citrus	6 fl oz	90	300	15
Veryfine Guava Strawberry	8 fl oz	120	100	30
Veryfine Pineapple Orange	8 fl oz	130	100	30
Wylers Lemonade	1 can (6 fl oz)	64	0	22
fruit punch	6 fl oz	87	26	55
orange grapefruit juice	8 fl oz	107	293	72
orange & apricot	8 fl oz	128	1450	50
pineapple & grapefruit	8 fl oz	117	88	115
pineapple & orange drink	8 fl oz	125	1320	56

FRUIT MIXED

CANNED

FOOD	PORTION	CAL	VIT A	VIT C
Chunky Mixed, Diet (S&W)	½ cup	40	200	12
Chunky Mixed, Natural Style (S&W)	½ cup	90	200	2
Chunky Mixed, Unsweetened (S&W)	½ cup	40	200	2
Fruit Cocktail (Hunt's)	4 oz	90	23	2
Fruit Cocktail, Diet (S&W)	½ cup	40	200	12
Fruit Cocktail, Natural Lite (S&W)	½ cup	60	200	9
Fruit Cocktail, Natural Style (S&W)	½ cup	90	200	2
Fruit Cocktail, Unsweetened (S&W)	½ cup	40	200	2

FOOD	PORTION	CAL	VIT A	VIT C
fruit cocktail in heavy syrup	½ cup	93	262	2
fruit cocktail in juice pack	½ cup	56	378	3
fruit cocktail in water pack	½ cup	40	305	3
fruit salad in heavy syrup	½ cup	94	646	3
fruit salad in juice pack	½ cup	62	744	4
fruit salad in light syrup	½ cup	73	541	3
fruit salad in water pack	½ cup	37	536	2
mixed fruit in heavy syrup	½ cup	92	248	88
tropical fruit salad in heavy syrup	½ cup	110	162	22
DRIED				
mixed	11 oz pkg	712	7155	11
FROZEN				
Mixed (Big Valley)	3.5 oz	45	750	90
Mixed Fruit (Birds Eye)	½ cup	120	300	27
mixed fruit, sweetened	1 cup	245	806	188

FRUIT SNACKS

FOOD	PORTION	CAL	VIT A	VIT C
Health Valley				
Bakes Apple	1 bar	100	4	3
Bakes Date	1 bar	100	5	3
Bakes Raisin	1 bar	100	5	4
Oat Bran Bakes Apricot	1 bar	100	1	1
Oat Bran Bakes Fig & Nut	1 bar	110	14	1
Oat Bran Jumbo Fruit Bar Almond & Date	1 bar	170	30	3
Oat Bran Jumbo Fruit Bars Raisin & Cinnamon	1 bar	160	3	7
Rice Bran Jumbo Fruit Bars Almond & Date	1 bar	160	117	4
Sunkist				
Fruit Flippits Cherry	0.8 oz	107	0	0
Fruit Flippits Strawberry	0.8 oz	107	0	0

FOOD	PORTION	CAL	VIT A	VIT C
Fruit Roll Apricot	1	76	102	1
Fruit Roll Cherry	1	75	11	1
Fruit Roll Grape	1	76	11	1
Fruit Roll Raspberry	1	75	17	1
Fruit Roll Strawberry	1	74	6	2
Fun Fruit Animals	0.9 oz	100	0	0
Fun Fruit Dinosaurs Strawberry	0.9 oz	100	0	0
Fun Fruit Spooky Fruit	1 pkg	100	0	0
Fun Fruit Strawberry	0.9 oz	100	0	0

GARLIC

clove	1	4	0	1

GELATIN

DRINKS

Orange Flavored Drinking Gelatin w/ Nutrasweet (Knox)	1 pkg	39	0	113

MIX
Jell-O

Apricot	½ cup	82	0	0
Black Cherry	½ cup	82	0	0
Black Raspberry	½ cup	82	0	0
Blackberry	½ cup	82	0	0
Concord Grape	½ cup	82	0	0
Lemon	½ cup	82	0	0
Lime	½ cup	82	0	0
Mixed Fruit	½ cup	82	0	0
Orange	½ cup	82	0	0
Wild Strawberry	½ cup	81	0	0
fruit flavored	½ cup	70	0	0
low calorie	½ cup	8	0	0

FOOD	PORTION	CAL	VIT A	VIT C

GIBLETS
(The vitamin A in giblets comes from animal sources.)

FOOD	PORTION	CAL	VIT A	VIT C
capon, simmered	1 cup (5 oz)	238	19236	13
chicken, floured & fried	1 cup (5 oz)	402	17298	13
chicken, simmered	1 cup (5 oz)	228	10774	12
turkey, simmered	1 cup (5 oz)	243	8753	3

GINGER

root, fresh	¼ cup	17	0	1
root, fresh	5 slices	8	0	1
root, fresh, sliced	¼ cup	17	0	1
root, fresh, sliced	5 slices	8	0	1

GINKGO NUTS

dried	1 oz	99	310	8
raw	1 oz	52	158	4

GIZZARDS
(The vitamin A in gizzards comes from animal sources.)

chicken, simmered	1 cup (5 oz)	222	273	2
turkey, simmered	1 cup (5 oz)	236	268	2

GOOSE
(The vitamin A in goose comes from animal sources.)

FRESH				
w/ skin, roasted	½ goose (1.7 lbs)	2362	541	0
w/ skin, roasted	6.6 oz	574	131	0

GOOSEBERRIES

fresh	1 cup	67	435	42
canned, in light syrup	½ cup	93	174	13

FOOD	PORTION	CAL	VIT A	VIT C

GRANOLA

BARS

FOOD	PORTION	CAL	VIT A	VIT C
New Trail Chocolate Covered Cookies and Creme	1	200	tr	tr
Quaker Chewy				
Chocolate Chip	1	128	0	0
Chunky Nut & Raisin	1	131	0	0
Cinnamon Raisin	1	128	0	0
Honey & Oats	1	125	0	0
Peanut Butter	1	128	0	0
Peanut Butter Chocolate Chip	1	131	0	0
Quaker Dipps				
Carmel Nut	1	148	0	0
Chocolate Chip	1	139	0	0
Chocolate Fudge	1	160	48	tr
Peanut Butter	1	170	29	tr
Peanut Butter Chocolate Chip	1	174	30	tr
CEREAL				
Quaker Sun Country 100% Natural With Raisins & Dates	¼ cup	123	0	0
Quaker Sun Country With Raisins	¼ cup	125	0	0

GRAPEFRUIT

CANNED

FOOD	PORTION	CAL	VIT A	VIT C
juice pack	½ cup	46	0	42
unsweetened	1 cup	93	18	72
water pack	½ cup	44	0	27
FRESH				
Dole	½	50	776	65
pink	½	37	318	47
pink sections	1 cup	69	595	88

FOOD	PORTION	CAL	VIT A	VIT C
red	½	37	318	47
red sections	1 cup	69	595	88
white	½	39	12	39
white sections	1 cup	76	23	77
JUICE				
frzn, as prep	1 cup	102	22	83
frzn, not prep	6 oz	302	65	248
sweetened	1 cup	116	0	67

GRAPES

FOOD	PORTION	CAL	VIT A	VIT C
CANNED				
Thompson Seedless In Heavy Syrup (S&W)	½ cup	94	81	1
Thompson Seedless Water Pack (S&W)	½ cup	48	81	1
FRESH				
grapes	10	36	35	5
JUICE				
S&W Concord Unsweetened	6 oz	100	0	1
bottled	1 cup	155	20	tr
frzn sweetened, as prep	1 cup	128	19	60
frzn sweetened, not prep	6 oz	386	58	180
grape drink	6 oz	84	2	64

GRAVY
(The vitamin A in gravy comes from animal sources.)

FOOD	PORTION	CAL	VIT A	VIT C
CANNED				
Bovril	1 heaping tsp	9	0	0
Marmite	1 heaping tsp	9	0	0
au jus	1 cup	38	0	2
beef	1 can (10 oz)	155	0	0
beef	1 cup	124	0	0
chicken	1 cup	189	880	0

FOOD	PORTION	CAL	VIT A	VIT C
mushroom	1 cup	120	0	0
turkey	1 cup	122	0	0
DRY				
Bournvita	2 heaping tsp	34	tr	0
Brown (Pillsbury)	¼ cup	15	0	0
Chicken (Pillsbury)	¼ cup	25	0	0
Home Style (Pillsbury)	¼ cup	15	0	0
Oil-Less Roux And Gravy Mix (Cajun King)	3.5 oz	394	242	12

GREAT NORTHERN BEANS

FOOD	PORTION	CAL	VIT A	VIT C
CANNED				
Green Giant	½ cup	80	0	0
Trappey's	½ cup	80	tr	tr
great northern	1 cup	300	3	3
DRIED				
cooked	1 cup	210	2	2

GREEN BEANS

FOOD	PORTION	CAL	VIT A	VIT C
CANNED				
Almondine (Green Giant)	½ cup	45	300	0
Cut (Green Giant)	½ cup	16	200	2
Cut Premium Blue Lake (S&W)	½ cup	20	300	5
Cut Water Pack (S&W)	½ cup	20	600	4
French (Green Giant)	½ cup	16	200	2
French Style Premium Blue Lake (S&W)	½ cup	20	300	5
Green Beans & Wax Beans (S&W)	½ cup	20	100	6
Kitchen Sliced (Green Giant)	½ cup	16	400	1
Whole Fancy Stringless (S&W)	½ cup	20	300	5
Whole Vertical Pack (S&W)	½ cup	20	300	5

FOOD	PORTION	CAL	VIT A	VIT C
FROZEN				
Cut (Birds Eye)	½ cup	25	500	9
Cut In Butter Sauce (Green Giant)	½ cup	30	200	2
Farm Fresh Whole (Birds Eye)	¾ cup	30	1000	12
French Cut (Birds Eye)	½ cup	25	400	9
French Green Beans In Sauce With Toasted Almonds (Birds Eye)	½ cup	50	400	9
Green Giant	½ cup	14	100	2
Harvest Fresh Cut (Green Giant)	½ cup	16	100	4
Italian (Birds Eye)	½ cup	30	400	15
One Serve In Butter Sauce (Green Giant)	1 pkg	60	300	tr
Polybag Cut (Birds Eye)	½ cup	25	500	9
Polybag Deluxe Whole (Birds Eye)	½ cup	20	400	9
Polybag French Cut (Birds Eye)	½ cup	25	500	9
Whole Deluxe (Birds Eye)	½ cup	45	500	21

GROUND-CHERRIES

FOOD	PORTION	CAL	VIT A	VIT C
fresh	½ cup	37	504	8

GUAVA

FOOD	PORTION	CAL	VIT A	VIT C
fresh	1	45	713	165
guava sauce	½ cup	43	337	174
JUICE				
Kern's Nectar	6 oz	110	500	27
Libby's Nectar	6 oz	110	200	54
Libby's Ripe Nectar	8 oz	140	200	72

FOOD	PORTION	CAL	VIT A	VIT C

HAM

(The vitamin A in ham dishes may come from either animal or plant sources.)

FOOD	PORTION	CAL	VIT A	VIT C
Carl Buddig	1 oz	50	0	0
canned (13% fat)	3 oz	192	0	12
canned, extra lean (4% fat)	3 oz	116	0	23
steak boneless, extra lean	1 oz	35	0	9

HAM DISHES

HOME RECIPE

FOOD	PORTION	CAL	VIT A	VIT C
croquettes	1 (3.1 oz)	217	206	tr
salad	½ cup	287	253	1

TAKE-OUT

FOOD	PORTION	CAL	VIT A	VIT C
sandwich w/ cheese	1	353	319	3

HAMBURGER

(The vitamin A in prepared hamburgers comes from both animal and plant sources.)

FOOD	PORTION	CAL	VIT A	VIT C
double patty w/ bun	1 reg	544	0	0
double patty w/ catsup, mayonnaise, onion, pickle tomato & bun	1 reg	649	371	3
double patty w/ catsup, cheese, mayonnaise, mustard, pickle, tomato & bun	1 lg	706	348	tr
double patty w/ catsup, mustard, mayonnaise, onion, pickle, tomato & bun	1 lg	540	102	1
double patty w/ catsup, mustard, onion, pickle & bun	1 reg	576	53	1
double patty w/ cheese & bun	1 reg	457	332	0
double patty w/ cheese & double bun	1 reg	461	276	0
double patty w/ cheese, catsup, mayonnaise, onion, pickle, tomato & bun	1 reg	416	398	2

FOOD	PORTION	CAL	VIT A	VIT C
single patty w/ bacon, catsup, cheese, mustard, onion, pickle & bun	1 lg	609	406	2
single patty w/ bun	1 lg	400	0	0
single patty w/ bun	1 reg	275	0	0
single patty w/ catsup, cheese, ham, mayonnaise, pickle, tomato & bun	1 lg	745	505	7
single patty w/ catsup, mustard, mayonnaise, onion, pickle, tomato & bun	1 reg	279	82	2
single patty w/ cheese & bun	1 lg	608	615	0
single patty w/ cheese & bun	1 reg	320	153	0
triple patty w/ catsup, mustard, pickle & bun	1 lg	693	158	1
triple patty w/ cheese & bun	1 lg	769	359	3

HEART

FOOD	PORTION	CAL	VIT A	VIT C
beef, simmered	3 oz	148	0	1
chicken, simmered	1 cup (5 oz)	268	41	3
lamb, braised	3 oz	158	0	6
turkey, simmered	1 cup (5 oz)	257	40	3

HERBS/SPICES

FOOD	PORTION	CAL	VIT A	VIT C
curry powder	1 tsp	6	20	tr
poultry seasoning	1 tsp	5	39	tr
pumpkin pie spice	1 tsp	6	4	tr

HERRING
(The vitamin A in herring comes from animal sources.)

FRESH				
atlantic, cooked	1 fillet (5 oz)	290	146	1
atlantic, cooked	3 oz	172	87	1

FOOD	PORTION	CAL	VIT A	VIT C
atlantic, raw	3 oz	134	80	1
READY-TO-USE				
atlantic kippered	1 fillet (1.4 oz)	87	51	tr

HONEY

honey	1 cup	1030	0	3
honey	1 tbsp	65	0	tr

HONEYDEW

cubed	1 cup	60	68	42
fresh	⅒	46	52	32

HOT DOG
(The vitamin A in prepared hot dogs comes mostly from animal sources, with a smaller amount from plant sources.)

TAKE-OUT				
corndog	1	460	207	0
w/ bun & chili	1	297	58	3
w/ bun, plain	1	242	0	tr

HUMMUS

hummus	1 cup	420	61	19
hummus	⅓ cup	140	20	6

ICE CREAM AND FROZEN DESSERTS
(The vitamin A in ice cream and frozen desserts comes from animal sources.)

Berry Berry Berry (Mocha Mix)	3.5 oz	209	6	2
Black Cherry Fat Free (Borden)	½ cup	90	0	0
Chocolate (Ultra Slim-Fast)	4 oz	100	750	9
Chocolate Fat Free (Borden)	½ cup	100	0	0

FOOD	PORTION	CAL	VIT A	VIT C
Chocolate Fudge (Ultra Slim-Fast)	4 oz	120	750	9
Dutch Chocolate (Mocha Mix)	3.5 oz	210	1	0
Fudge Bar (Ultra Slim-Fast)	1	90	500	6
Heavenly Hash (Mocha Mix)	3.5 oz	244	13	0
Mocha Almond Fudge (Mocha Mix)	3.5 oz	229	tr	0
Neapolitan (Mocha Mix)	3.5 oz	208	tr	tr
Orange & Cream Pop (Haagen-Dazs)	1	130	300	6
Peach (Mocha Mix)	3.5 oz	198	68	0
Peach (Ultra Slim-Fast)	4 oz	100	750	9
Peach Fat Free (Borden)	½ cup	90	0	0
Pralines And Caramel (Ultra Slim-Fast)	4 oz	120	750	9
Strawberry Fat Free (Borden)	½ cup	90	0	0
Strawberry Swirl (Mocha Mix)	3.5 oz	209	2	1
Toasted Almond (Mocha Mix)	3.5 oz	229	0	0
Vanilla (Mocha Mix)	3.5 oz	209	0	0
Vanilla (Ultra Slim-Fast)	4 oz	90	750	9
Vanilla Chocolate Sandwich (Ultra Slim-Fast)	1	140	500	6
Vanilla Cookie Crunch Bar (Ultra Slim-Fast)	1	90	500	6
Vanilla Fat Free (Borden)	½ cup	90	0	0
Vanilla Fudge Cookie (Ultra Slim-Fast)	4 oz	110	750	9
Vanilla Oatmeal Sandwich (Ultra Slim-Fast)	1	150	500	6
Vanilla Sandwich (Ultra Slim-Fast)	1	140	500	6
french vanilla soft serve	1 cup	377	794	1
french vanilla soft serve	½ gal	3014	6353	7

FOOD	PORTION	CAL	VIT A	VIT C
vanilla 10% fat	1 cup	269	543	1
vanilla 10% fat	½ gal	2153	4341	6
vanilla 16% fat	1 cup	349	879	1
vanilla 16% fat	½ gal	2805	7199	5
vanilla ice milk	1 cup	184	214	1
vanilla ice milk	½ gal	1469	1708	6
vanilla ice milk soft serve	1 cup	223	175	1
vanilla ice milk soft serve	½ gal	1787	1400	9
TAKE-OUT				
cone, vanilla ice milk soft serve	1 (4.6 oz)	164	211	1
sundae, caramel	1 (5.4 oz)	303	263	3
sundae, hot fudge	1 (5.4 oz)	284	221	2
sundae, strawberry	1 (5.4 oz)	269	222	2

ICE CREAM CONES AND CUPS

sugar cone	1	40	0	0
wafer cone	1	17	0	0

ICES AND ICE POPS
(The vitamin A in ices and ice pops comes mainly from plant sources, with a small amount from animal sources when milk or cream is added.)

Dole Fruit N' Cream Bar				
Peach	1 bar	90	200	15
Raspberry	1 bar	90	49	5
Strawberry	1 bar	90	11	6
Dole Fruit N' Juice Bar				
Pineapple	1 bar	70	17	4
Raspberry	1 bar	70	11	2
Strawberry	1 bar	70	6	1
Dole Sorbet				
Mandarin Orange	4 oz	110	312	25

FOOD	PORTION	CAL	VIT A	VIT C
Dole Sorbet *(cont.)*				
Pineapple	4 oz	110	12	6
Strawberry	4 oz	100	6	4
Dole SunTops				
Grape	1 bar	40	2	2
Lemonade	1 bar	40	2	2
Orange	1 bar	40	32	1

JACKFRUIT

fresh	3½ oz	70	tr	9

JAM/JELLY/PRESERVES

cherry jam	3½ oz	250	0	1

JAVA PLUM

fresh	1 cup	82	5	19
fresh	3	5	0	1

JEW'S EAR

pepeao, dried	½ cup	36	0	tr
pepeao, raw sliced	1 cup	25	0	1

JUJUBE

fresh	3½ oz	105	tr	58

KALE

FRESH				
Dole, chopped	½ cup	17	3026	41
chopped, cooked	½ cup	21	4810	27
chopped, raw	½ cup	21	3026	41
scotch, chopped, cooked	½ cup	18	1296	34
FROZEN				
chopped, cooked	½ cup	20	4130	16

FOOD	PORTION	CAL	VIT A	VIT C
KIDNEY				
(The vitamin A in kidney comes from animal sources.)				
beef, simmered	3 oz	122	1055	1
lamb, braised	3 oz	117	387	10
veal, braised	3 oz	139	569	7
KIDNEY BEANS				
CANNED				
Goya Spanish Style	7.5 oz	140	444	3
Green Giant Dark Red	½ cup	90	0	0
Green Giant Light Red	½ cup	90	0	0
Hunt's Red	4 oz	100	tr	1
Trappey's New Orleans Style	½ cup	100	tr	tr
Van Camp's Dark Red	1 cup	182	0	0
Van Camp's Light Red	1 cup	184	0	0
Van Camp's New Orleans Style Red	1 cup	178	0	0
kidney beans	1 cup	208	0	3
red	1 cup	216	0	3
DRIED				
california red, cooked	1 cup	219	5	2
cooked	1 cup	225	0	2
red, cooked	1 cup	225	0	2
royal red, cooked	1 cup	218	5	2
SPROUTS				
cooked	1 lb	152	8	162
raw	½ cup	27	2	36
KIWIS				
Dole	2	90	136	143
fresh	1 med	46	133	75

FOOD	PORTION	CAL	VIT A	VIT C
KOHLRABI				
FRESH				
raw, sliced	½ cup	19	25	43
cooked, sliced	½ cup	24	29	44
KUMQUATS				
fresh	1	12	57	7
LAMB DISHES				

(The vitamin A in lamb dishes comes from both animal and plant sources.)

FOOD	PORTION	CAL	VIT A	VIT C
TAKE-OUT				
curry	¾ cup	345	145	3
moussaka	5.6 oz	312	330	6
stew	¾ cup	124	4265	20
LAMB'S-QUARTERS				
fresh, chopped, cooked	½ cup	29	8730	33
LEEKS				
DRIED				
freeze dried	1 tbsp	1	1	tr
FRESH				
chopped, cooked	¼ cup	8	12	1
cooked	1 (4.4 oz)	38	57	5
raw	1 (4.4 oz)	76	110	15
raw, chopped	¼ cup	16	25	3
LEMON				
lemon	1 med	22	32	83
peel	1 tbsp	0	3	8
wedge	1	5	8	21
JUICE				
bottled	1 tbsp	3	2	4

FOOD	PORTION	CAL	VIT A	VIT C
fresh	1 tbsp	4	3	7
frzn	1 tbsp	3	2	5

LEMON CURD
(The vitamin A in lemon curd comes from animal ingredients like egg and from plant sources.)

FOOD	PORTION	CAL	VIT A	VIT C
lemon curd made w/ egg	2 tsp	29	70	1
lemon curd made w/ starch	2 tsp	28	5	0

LENTILS

FOOD	PORTION	CAL	VIT A	VIT C
CANNED				
Health Valley Fast Menu Hearty Lentils Garden Vegetables	7½ oz	150	5000	4
Health Valley Fast Menu Organic Lentils With Tofu Weiners	7½ oz	170	5000	1
dried, cooked	1 cup	231	15	3
sprouts, raw	½ cup	40	17	6

LETTUCE

FOOD	PORTION	CAL	VIT A	VIT C
Dole Butter Lettuce	1 head	21	1581	13
Dole Iceberg	⅙ med head	20	166	3
Dole Leaf, shredded	1½ cup	12	1596	15
Dole Romaine, shredded	1½ cups	18	2184	20
bibb	1 head (6 oz)	21	1581	13
boston	1 head (6 oz)	21	1581	13
boston	2 leaves	2	146	1
iceberg	1 head (19 oz)	70	1779	21
iceberg	1 leaf	3	66	1
looseleaf, shredded	½ cup	5	532	5
romaine, shredded	½ cup	4	728	7

FOOD	PORTION	CAL	VIT A	VIT C
LIMA BEANS				
CANNED				
S&W Small Fancy	½ cup	80	100	6
Trappey's Baby Green	½ cup	90	100	tr
Trappey's Baby White	½ cup	90	100	tr
large	1 cup	191	0	0
lima beans	½ cup	93	214	11
DRIED				
baby, cooked	1 cup	229	0	0
cooked	½ cup	104	315	9
large, cooked	1 cup	217	0	0
FROZEN				
Birds Eye, Baby	½ cup	130	200	18
Birds Eye, Fordhook	½ cup	100	200	18
Green Giant Harvest Fresh	½ cup	80	0	2
Green Giant, In Butter Sauce	½ cup	100	100	4
cooked	½ cup	94	150	5
fordhook, cooked	½ cup	85	162	1
LIME				
FRESH				
lime	1	20	7	20
JUICE				
bottled	1 tbsp	3	3	1
fresh	1 tbsp	4	2	5
LIQUOR/LIQUEUR				
bloody mary	5 oz	116	508	20
bourbon & soda	4 oz	105	0	0
coffee liqueur	1½ oz	174	0	0
daiquiri	2 oz	111	2	1
gin	1½ oz	110	0	0

FOOD	PORTION	CAL	VIT A	VIT C
gin & tonic	7.5 oz	171	2	1
manhattan	2 oz	128	0	0
pina colada	4½ oz	262	3	7
rum	1½ oz	97	0	0
screwdriver	7 oz	174	133	67
sloe gin fizz	2½ oz	132	5	1
tequila sunrise	5½ oz	189	166	13
tom collins	7½ oz	121	2	4
vodka	1½ oz	97	0	0
whiskey	1½ oz	105	0	0
whiskey sour	3 oz	123	7	11
whiskey sour mix, as prep	3.6 oz	169	5	1
whiskey sour mix, not prep	1 pkg (0.6 oz)	64	5	1

LIVER
(The vitamin A in liver comes from animal sources.)

beef, braised	3 oz	137	30327	19
beef, pan-fried	3 oz	184	30689	19
chicken, stewed	1 cup (5 oz)	219	22925	22
lamb, braised	3 oz	187	21203	3
lamb, fried	3 oz	202	22098	11
pork, braised	3 oz	141	15297	20
turkey, simmered	1 cup (5 oz)	237	17614	3
veal, braised	3 oz	140	22851	26
veal, fried	3 oz	208	15978	18

LOGANBERRIES

frzn	1 cup	80	52	23

LOTUS

root, raw, sliced	10 slices	45	0	36

FOOD	PORTION	CAL	VIT A	VIT C
root, sliced, cooked	10 slices	59	0	24
seeds, dried	1 oz	94	14	0

LUNCHEON MEATS/COLD CUTS
(The vitamin A in luncheon meats comes from animal sources; the exception is the sandwich, which contains some plant sources.)

FOOD	PORTION	CAL	VIT A	VIT C
Carl Buddig Beef	1 oz	40	0	0
Carl Buddig Corned Beef	1 oz	40	0	0
Carl Buddig Pastrami	1 oz	40	0	0
braunschweiger, pork	1 oz	102	3984	8
braunschweiger, pork	1 slice (2½ × ¼ in)	65	2529	2
liver cheese, pork	1 oz	86	4957	1
TAKE-OUT				
submarine w/ salami, ham, cheese, lettuce, tomato, onion & oil	1	456	425	12

LYCHEES

FOOD	PORTION	CAL	VIT A	VIT C
fresh	1	6	0	7

MACADAMIA NUTS

FOOD	PORTION	CAL	VIT A	VIT C
oil roasted	1 oz	204	3	0

MACKEREL
(The vitamin A in mackerel comes from plant sources.)

FOOD	PORTION	CAL	VIT A	VIT C
CANNED				
jack	1 can (12.7 oz)	563	1567	3
jack	1 cup	296	825	2
FRESH				
atlantic, cooked	3 oz	223	153	tr
atlantic, raw	3 oz	174	140	tr

FOOD	PORTION	CAL	VIT A	VIT C

MALTED MILK
(The vitamin A in prepared malted milk comes from animal sources; in malted milk powder, the vitamin A comes from a plant source.)

chocolate, as prep w/ milk	1 cup	229	326	3
chocolate flavor, powder	3 heaping tsp (¾ oz)	79	19	tr
natural flavor, as prep w/ milk	1 cup	237	369	3
natural flavor, powder	3 heaping tsp (¾ oz)	87	61	1

MAMMY-APPLE
fresh	1	431	1946	118

MANGO
fresh	1	135	8060	57
JUICE				
Kern's Nectar	6 oz	110	1000	27
Libby's Nectar	6 oz	110	1750	27

MARGARINE
(The vitamin A in margarine comes from plant sources.)

REDUCED CALORIE				
diet	1 cup	800	7672	tr
diet	1 tsp	17	159	tr
REGULAR				
corn	1 stick (4 oz)	815	3750	tr
corn	1 tsp	34	155	tr
salted	1 stick (4 oz)	815	3750	tr
salted	1 tsp	39	155	tr
unsalted	1 stick (4 oz)	809	3750	tr
unsalted	1 tsp	34	155	tr
SOFT				
corn	1 cup	1626	7507	tr

FOOD	PORTION	CAL	VIT A	VIT C
corn	1 tsp	34	155	tr
safflower	1 cup	1626	2254	tr
safflower	1 tsp	34	21	tr
soybean, salted	1 cup	1626	7507	tr
soybean, salted	1 tsp	34	155	tr
soybean, unsalted	1 cup	1626	7507	tr
soybean, unsalted	1 tsp	34	155	tr
tub, salted	1 cup	1626	7507	tr
tub, salted	1 tsp	34	155	tr
tub, unsalted	1 cup	1626	7507	tr
tub, unsalted	1 tsp	34	155	tr
SQUEEZE soybean & cottonseed	1 tsp	34	155	tr

MARSHMALLOW

FOOD	PORTION	CAL	VIT A	VIT C
Marshmallow Fluff	1 heaping tsp (18 g)	59	tr	tr
marshmallow	1 oz	90	0	0

MAYONNAISE TYPE SALAD DRESSING
(The vitamin A in mayonnaise comes mostly from animal sources.)

FOOD	PORTION	CAL	VIT A	VIT C
REGULAR home recipe	1 cup	400	1048	2
home recipe	1 tbsp	25	66	tr

MEAT SUBSTITUTES
(The vitamin A in meat substitutes comes mostly from plant sources.)

FOOD	PORTION	CAL	VIT A	VIT C
simulated sausage	1 link (25 g)	64	160	0
simulated sausage	1 patty (38 g)	97	243	0

FOOD	PORTION	CAL	VIT A	VIT C

MELON

FROZEN

Mixed Balls (Big Valley)	3.5 oz	35	1250	21
melon balls	1 cup	55	3096	11

MILK

(The vitamin A in milk comes from animal sources.)

CANNED

condensed, sweetened	1 cup	982	1004	8
condensed, sweetened	1 oz	123	125	1
evaporated	½ cup	169	306	2
evaporated skim	½ cup	99	500	2

DRIED

Lactose Reduced, as prep (Nutra/Balance)	8 oz	80	500	1
Sanalac, as prep	8 oz	80	100	1
buttermilk	1 tbsp	25	14	tr
nonfat, instantized	1 pkg (3.2 oz)	244	2157	5

LIQUID, LOWFAT

1%	1 cup	102	500	2
1%	1 qt	409	2000	9
1% protein fortified	1 cup	119	500	3
1% protein fortified	1 qt	477	2000	11
2%	1 cup	121	500	2
2%	1 qt	485	2000	9
Borden Acidophilus 1%	8 fl oz	100	500	2
Borden Golden Churn Lowfat Buttermilk	8 fl oz	120	200	2
Borden Hi-Protein 2%	8 fl oz	140	500	4
CalciMilk	8 fl oz	102	500	2
Lactaid 1%	8 fl oz	102	500	2
Viva 2%	8 fl oz	120	500	2

FOOD	PORTION	CAL	VIT A	VIT C
buttermilk	1 cup	99	81	2
buttermilk	1 qt	396	323	10
LIQUID, REGULAR				
Borden	8 fl oz	150	200	2
Borden Hi-Calcium	8 fl oz	150	200	2
Farmland Cholesterol Reduced	8 oz	150	200	2
goat	1 cup	168	451	3
goat	1 qt	672	1806	13
human	1 cup	171	593	12
indian buffalo	1 cup	236	434	5
mare	3½ oz	49	tr	15
sheep	1 cup	264	360	10
whole	1 cup	150	307	2
LIQUID, SKIM				
Borden	8 fl oz	90	500	2
Borden Skim-Line	8 fl oz	100	500	4
Farmland Skim Plus	8 fl oz	100	500	4
Lactaid Nonfat	8 fl oz	86	500	2
Viva	8 fl oz	100	500	4
skim	1 cup	86	500	2
skim	1 qt	342	2000	10
skim, protein fortified	1 cup	100	500	3
skim, protein fortified	1 qt	400	2000	11

MILK DRINKS
(The vitamin A in milk drinks comes from animal sources.)

FOOD	PORTION	CAL	VIT A	VIT C
Chocolate Lowfat Dutch Brand (Borden)	8 fl oz	180	500	2
Chocolate Milk (Meadow Gold)	8 fl oz	210	200	2
Chocolate Milk 1% (Lactaid)	8 fl oz	158	500	2
Chocolate Milk 2% (Hershey)	1 cup	190	500	2

FOOD	PORTION	CAL	VIT A	VIT C
Quik Chocolate, as prep w/ 2% milk (Nestle)	8 oz	210	500	2
Quik Chocolate, as prep w/ skim milk (Nestle)	8 oz	170	500	2
Quik Chocolate, as prep w/ whole milk (Nestle)	8 oz	230	300	2
Quik Lite Ready To Drink Chocolate Lowfat (Nestle)	8 oz	130	500	2
Quik Ready to Drink Chocolate (Nestle)	8 oz	230	200	1
Quik Ready to Drink Strawberry (Nestlo)	8 oz	230	200	2
Quik Strawberry, as prep w/ 2% milk (Nestle)	8 oz	200	500	2
Quik Strawberry, as prep w/ skim milk (Nestle)	8 oz	160	500	2
Quik Strawberry, as prep w/ whole milk (Nestle)	8 oz	220	300	2
Quik Sugar Free Chocolate, as prep w/ 2% milk (Nestle)	8 oz	140	500	1
Quik Syrup Chocolate, as prep w/ 2% milk (Nestle)	8 oz	220	500	2
Quik Syrup Chocolate, as prep w/ skim milk (Nestle)	8 oz	220	300	2
Quik Syrup Chocolate, as prep w/ whole milk (Nestle)	8 oz	240	300	2
Quik Syrup Strawberry, as prep w/ 2% milk (Nestle)	8 oz	220	500	2
Quik Syrup Strawberry, as prep w/ skim milk (Nestle)	8 oz	180	500	2
Quik Syrup Strawberry, as prep w/ whole milk (Nestle)	8 oz	240	300	2
Whole Chocolate Milk (Hershey)	8 oz	210	200	2
chocolate milk	1 cup	208	302	2

FOOD	PORTION	CAL	VIT A	VIT C
chocolate milk	1 qt	833	1210	9
chocolate milk 1%	1 cup	158	500	2
chocolate milk 1%	1 qt	630	2000	9
chocolate milk 2%	1 cup	179	500	2
strawberry flavor milk, as prep w/ whole milk	9 oz	234	308	2

MILK SUBSTITUTES

First Alternative	8 fl oz	80	500	2
Vegelicious	8 fl oz	100	500	6
imitation milk	1 cup	150	0	0
imitation milk	1 qt	600	0	0

MILKSHAKE
(The vitamin A in milkshakes comes from animal sources.)

chocolate	10 oz	360	263	1
chocolate thick shake	10.6 oz	356	258	0
strawberry	10 oz	319	340	2
vanilla	10 oz	314	368	2
vanilla thick shake	11 oz	350	357	0

MISO

miso	½ cup	284	120	0

MOLASSES

blackstrap	2 tbsp	85	0	0
molasses	2 tbsp	85	0	0

MOTH BEANS

DRIED
cooked	1 cup	207	17	2

FOOD	PORTION	CAL	VIT A	VIT C

MOUSSE
(The vitamin A in mousse comes from animal ingredients like cream.)

FROZEN
Sara Lee

FOOD	PORTION	CAL	VIT A	VIT C
Chocolate	1 slice (2.7 oz)	260	400	1
Chocolate Light	1 (3 oz)	170	300	0

MIX
JELL-O

FOOD	PORTION	CAL	VIT A	VIT C
Chocolate Fudge Rich And Luscious	½ cup	143	82	1
Chocolate Rich And Luscious	½ cup	145	81	1

MUFFIN
(The vitamin A in muffins comes from animal ingredients like milk and eggs and from plant sources like blueberries.)

FROZEN

FOOD	PORTION	CAL	VIT A	VIT C
Almond & Date Oat Bran Fancy Fruit (Health Valley)	1	180	54	2
Apple Oat Bran (Sara Lee)	1	190	1250	2
Apple Spice (Healthy Choice)	1 (2.5 oz)	190	100	5
Apple Spice (Sara Lee)	1	220	1250	5
Blueberry (Healthy Choice)	1 (2.5 oz)	190	100	4
Blueberry (Sara Lee)	1	200	1250	1
Blueberry Free & Light (Sara Lee)	1	120	1250	1
Cheese Streusel (Sara Lee)	1	220	100	0
Golden Corn (Sara Lee)	1	240	1250	0
Oat Bran (Sara Lee)	1	210	1250	1
Oat Bran Fancy Fruit Blueberry (Health Valley)	1	140	36	5
Oat Bran Fancy Fruit Raisin (Health Valley)	1	180	60	7
Raisin Bran (Sara Lee)	1	220	1250	2

FOOD	PORTION	CAL	VIT A	VIT C
Rice Bran Fancy Fruit Raisin (Health Valley)	1	210	2	5
HOME RECIPE				
blueberry, as prep with 2% milk	1 (2 oz)	163	81	1
blueberry, as prep with whole milk	1 (2 oz)	165	63	1
corn, as prep w/ 2% milk	1 (2 oz)	180	137	tr
corn, as prep w/ whole milk	1 (2 oz)	183	118	tr
plain, as prep w/ 2% milk	1 (2 oz)	169	80	tr
plain, as prep w/ whole milk	1 (2 oz)	172	61	tr
wheat bran, as prep w/ 2% milk	1 (2 oz)	161	478	5
wheat bran, as prep w/ whole milk	1 (2 oz)	164	459	5
MIX				
corn	1 (1.75 oz)	160	105	tr
wheat bran, as prep	1 (1¾ oz)	138	51	0
READY-TO-EAT				
toaster type, blueberry	1	103	105	0
toaster type, corn	1	114	32	0
toaster type, wheat bran w/ raisins	1 (36 g)	106	64	0

MULBERRIES

FOOD	PORTION	CAL	VIT A	VIT C
fresh	1 cup	61	35	51

MUNG BEANS

FOOD	PORTION	CAL	VIT A	VIT C
DRIED				
cooked	1 cup	213	48	2
SPROUTS				
canned	½ cup	8	14	tr
cooked	½ cup	13	8	7
raw	½ cup	16	11	7

FOOD	PORTION	CAL	VIT A	VIT C
MUNGO BEANS				
DRIED				
cooked	1 cup	190	56	2
MUSHROOMS				
CANNED				
Mushrooms (B in B)	¼ cup	12	0	0
Mushrooms With Garlic (B in B)	¼ cup	12	0	0
Oriental Straw Mushrooms (Green Giant)	¼ cup	12	0	0
Pieces and Stems (Green Giant)	¼ cup	12	0	0
Sliced (Green Giant)	¼ cup	12	0	0
Whole (Green Giant)	¼ cup	12	0	0
chanterelle	3½ oz	12	1	3
FRESH				
enoki, raw	1 (4 in)	2	0	1
raw	1 (½ oz)	5	0	1
raw sliced	½ cup	9	0	1
cooked shiitake	4 (2.5 oz)	40	0	tr
sliced, cooked	½ cup	21	0	3
whole, cooked	1 (0.4 oz)	3	0	1
MUSTARD				
yellow ready-to-use	1 tsp	5	0	0
MUSTARD GREENS				
FRESH				
chopped, cooked	½ cup	11	2122	18
raw, chopped	½ cup	7	1484	20
FROZEN				
chopped, cooked	½ cup	14	3352	10

FOOD	PORTION	CAL	VIT A	VIT C

NATTO
| natto | ½ cup | 187 | 0 | 11 |

NAVY BEANS
CANNED
Trappey's	½ cup	90	tr	tr
Trappey's Jalapeno	½ cup	90	tr	tr
navy	1 cup	296	4	2
DRIED
| cooked | 1 cup | 259 | 3 | 2 |

NECTARINE
| fresh | 1 | 67 | 1001 | 7 |

NOODLES
(The vitamin A in noodles comes from animal ingredients
like egg and from plant sources like spinach.)

DRY
Egg (Golden Grain)	2 oz	210	0	0
cellophane	1 cup	492	0	0
chow mein	1 cup	237	38	0
egg	1 cup (38 g)	145	23	0
egg, cooked	1 cup	212	32	0
spinach/egg	1 cup	145	120	0
spinach/egg, cooked	1 cup	211	165	0

DRY MIX
Lipton Noodles and Sauce
Alfredo	½ cup	131	39	0
Beef	½ cup	120	0	1
Butter	½ cup	142	81	1
Butter and Herb	½ cup	136	71	0
Carbonara Alfredo	1/2 cup	126	61	1
Cheese	½ cup	136	61	0

FOOD	PORTION	CAL	VIT A	VIT C
Chicken	½ cup	125	33	0
Chicken Broccoli	½ cup	124	42	2
Creamy Chicken	½ cup	125	1069	tr
Parmesan	½ cup	138	128	0
Romanoff	½ cup	136	74	0
Sour Cream and Chive	½ cup	142	69	0
Stroganoff	½ cup	110	160	0
Tomato Alfredo	½ cup	126	1380	1
Minute Microwave Chicken Flavored	½ cup	157	840	1
Minute Microwave Parmesan	½ cup	178	198	tr
Ultra Slim-Fast Noodles & Alfredo Sauce	2.3 oz	240	750	18
Ultra Slim-Fast Noodles & Beef	2.3 oz	230	750	18
Ultra Slim-Fast Noodles & Cheese	2.3 oz	230	750	18
Ultra Slim-Fast Noodles & Chicken Sauce	2.3 oz	220	750	18
Ultra Slim-Fast Noodles & Tomato Herb Sauce	2.3 oz	220	750	18
TAKE-OUT noodle pudding	½ cup	132	260	1

NUTRITIONAL SUPPLEMENTS
(The vitamin A in nutritional supplements comes from animal sources like milk and plant sources.)

DIET				
Dynatrim Dutch Chocolate, as prep w/ 1% milk	8 oz	220	1750	21
Dynatrim Strawberry Royale, as prep w/ 1% milk	8 oz	220	1750	21
Dynatrim Vanilla, as prep w/ 1% milk	8 oz	220	1750	21

FOOD	PORTION	CAL	VIT A	VIT C
Figurines				
Chocolate	1 bar	100	500	9
Chocolate Caramel	1 bar	100	500	9
Chocolate Peanut Butter	1 bar	100	500	9
S'Mores	1 bar	100	500	9
Vanilla	1 bar	100	500	9
Slim-Fast Nutrition Bar Dutch Chocolate	1	130	1750	21
Slim-Fast Nutrition Bar Peanut Butter	1	140	1750	21
Slim-Fast Powder				
Chocolate Malt, as prep w/ skim milk	8 oz	190	1750	21
Chocolate, as prep w/ skim milk	8 oz	190	1750	21
Strawberry, as prep w/ skim milk	8 oz	190	1750	21
Vanilla, as prep w/ skim milk	8 oz	190	1750	21
Ultra Slim-Fast				
Cafe Mocha, as prep w/ skim milk	8 oz	200	1750	21
Chocolate Royale, as prep w/ skim milk	8 oz	200	1750	21
Crunch Bar Cocoa Almond	1	110	750	9
Crunch Bar Cocoa Raspberry	1	100	750	9
Crunch Bar Vanilla Almond	1	110	750	9
Dutch Chocolate, as prep w/ water	8 oz	220	1750	21
French Vanilla, as prep w/ skim milk	8 oz	190	1750	21
French Vanilla, as prep w/ water	8 oz	220	1750	21

FOOD	PORTION	CAL	VIT A	VIT C
Fruit Juice Mix, as prep w/ fruit juice	8 oz	200	1750	21
Pina Colada, as prep w/ skim milk	8 oz	180	1750	21
Ready-to-Drink Chocolate Royale	11 oz	230	1750	21
Ready-to-Drink Chocolate Royale	12 oz	250	1750	21
Ready-to-Drink French Vanilla	11 oz	220	1750	21
Ready-to-Drink French Vanilla	12 oz	230	1750	21
Ready-to-Drink Strawberry Supreme	12 oz	220	1750	21
Strawberry Supreme, as prep w/ water	8 oz	190	1750	21
Strawberry, as prep w/ skim milk	8 oz	220	1750	21

NUTS MIXED

FOOD	PORTION	CAL	VIT A	VIT C
Tasty Mix (Guy's)	1 oz	130	200	4
dry roasted w/ peanuts	1 oz	169	4	tr
dry roasted w/ peanuts, salted	1 oz	169	4	tr
oil roasted w/ peanuts	1 oz	175	6	tr
oil roasted w/ peanuts, salted	1 oz	175	6	tr
oil roasted w/o peanuts	1 oz	175	6	tr
oil roasted w/o peanuts, salted	1 oz	175	6	tr

OHELOBERRIES

FOOD	PORTION	CAL	VIT A	VIT C
fresh	1 cup	39	1162	8

OIL

FOOD	PORTION	CAL	VIT A	VIT C
Wesson Canola	1 tbsp	120	0	0

FOOD	PORTION	CAL	VIT A	VIT C
Wesson Corn	1 tbsp	120	0	0
Wesson Lite Cooking Spray	.5 sec spray	0	0	0
Wesson Olive	1 tbsp	120	0	0
Wesson Sunflower	1 tbsp	120	0	0
Wesson Vegetable	1 tbsp	120	0	0

OKRA

FOOD	PORTION	CAL	VIT A	VIT C
FRESH				
raw	8 pods	36	627	20
raw, sliced	½ cup	19	330	11
sliced, cooked	½ cup	25	460	13
sliced, cooked	8 pods	27	489	14
FROZEN				
Breaded Okra (Ore Ida)	3 oz	170	300	1
sliced, cooked	1 pkg (10 oz)	94	1311	31
sliced, cooked	½ cup	34	473	11

OLIVES

FOOD	PORTION	CAL	VIT A	VIT C
California Ripe	3 sm	4	403	0
Ripe Extra Large (S&W)	3.5 oz	163	200	4
Ripe Pitted Large (S&W)	3.5 oz	163	200	4
Spanish Green (Tee Pee)	2 oz	98	tr	tr
green	3 extra lg	15	40	0
green	4 med	15	40	0
ripe	1 colossal	12	53	tr
ripe	1 jumbo	7	29	tr
ripe	1 lg	5	18	0
ripe	1 sm	4	13	0

ONION

FOOD	PORTION	CAL	VIT A	VIT C
DRIED				
flakes	1 tbsp	16	0	4

FOOD	PORTION	CAL	VIT A	VIT C
FRESH				
Antioch Farms Vidalia	1 med	60	tr	12
Dole	1 med	60	0	11
Dole Green Onions, chopped	1 tbsp	2	300	3
chopped, cooked	½ cup	47	0	6
raw, chopped	1 tbsp	4	0	1
raw, chopped	½ cup	30	0	5
scallions, raw, chopped	1 tbsp	2	23	1
scallions, raw, sliced	½ cup	16	193	9
FROZEN				
chopped, cooked	1 tbsp	4	5	tr
chopped, cooked	½ cup	30	36	3
rings	7 (2.5 oz)	285	158	1
rings, cooked	2 (0.7 oz)	81	45	tr
whole, cooked	3½ oz	28	21	5
TAKE-OUT				
rings, breaded & fried	8 to 9	275	8	tr

ORANGE

FOOD	PORTION	CAL	VIT A	VIT C
CANNED				
Mandarin (Empress)	5.5 oz	100	2250	24
Mandarin Selected Sections In Heavy Syrup (S&W)	½ cup	76	200	6
Mandarin Unsweetened (S&W)	½ cup	28	400	18
Mandarin From Japan (Empress)	5.5 oz	35	750	21
Mandarin Natural Style (S&W)	½ cup	60	200	12
Pineapple Mandarin Segments (Dole)	½ cup	60	100	6
FRESH				
Dole	1	50	96	78
california valencia	1	59	278	59
california navel	1	65	256	80

FOOD	PORTION	CAL	VIT A	VIT C
florida	1	69	302	68
peel	1 tbsp	6	25	8
sections	1 cup	85	369	96
JUICE				
Kool-Aid Koolers	1 (8.45 oz)	115	11	6
Sippin' Pak 100% Pure	8.45 fl oz	110	100	60
Tang Breakfast Crystals Sugar Free, as prep	6 oz	5	500	60
Tang Breakfast Crystals, as prep	6 oz	86	500	60
Tang Fruit Box	8.45 oz	127	23	60
Tree Top	6 oz	90	200	66
Veryfine 100%	8 oz	121	400	84
Veryfine Orange Drink	8 oz	140	200	30
canned	1 cup	104	432	86
chilled	1 cup	110	194	82
fresh	1 cup	111	496	124
frzn, as prep	1 cup	112	194	97
frzn, not prep	6 oz	339	589	294
mandarin orange	3½ oz	47	tr	32
orange drink	6 oz	94	33	64

ORIENTAL FOOD

(The vitamin A in Oriental food comes from animal ingredients like beef and plant sources like vegetables.)

CANNED				
La Choy Bi-Pack				
Beef Pepper	¾ cup	80	350	21
Chow Mein Chicken	¾ cup	80	100	15
Chow Mein Pork	¾ cup	80	150	12
Chow Mein Shrimp	¾ cup	70	100	15
Sweet & Sour Chicken	¾ cup	120	400	15

FOOD	PORTION	CAL	VIT A	VIT C
Teriyaki Chicken	¾ cup	85	200	12
La Choy Dinner Chow Mein Chicken	¾ pkg	300	150	3
La Choy Entree				
Beef Pepper Oriental	¾ cup	100	450	9
Chow Mein Beef	¾ cup	40	150	2
Chow Mein Chicken	¾ cup	70	150	3
Chow Mein Meatless	¾ cup	25	100	5
Chow Mein Shrimp	¾ cup	35	100	6
Sweet And Sour Chicken	¾ cup	240	350	4
Sweet And Sour Pork	¾ cup	250	125	4
chow mein chicken	1 cup	95	150	tr
FRESH				
egg roll wrapper	1	83	4	0
wonton wrappers	1	23	1	0
FROZEN				
Birds Eye Chicken Teriyaki Easy Recipe, not prep	½ pkg	160	2250	15
Birds Eye Chinese Stir Fry Internationals, not prep	3.3 oz	35	750	12
Japanese Stir Fry International, not prep	3.3 oz	30	400	15
Birds Eye Oriental Beef Easy Recipe, not prep	½ pkg	100	750	54
Chun King				
Beef Pepper Oriental	13 oz	319	1500	18
Chicken Chow Mein	13 oz	370	500	4
Fried Rice With Chicken	8 oz	260	500	6
Fried Rice With Pork	8 oz	270	750	4
Imperial Chicken	13 oz	300	1250	9
Sweet & Sour Pork	13 oz	400	1500	12
Healthy Choice Chicken Chow Mein	8.5 oz	220	440	4

FOOD	PORTION	CAL	VIT A	VIT C
La Choy				
Restaurant Style Egg Roll, Pork	1 (3 oz)	150	300	18
Restaurant Style Egg Roll, Shrimp	1 (3 oz)	130	300	6
Restaurant Style Egg Roll, Almond Chicken	1 (3 oz)	120	400	6
Restaurant Style Egg Roll, Sweet & Sour Chicken	1 (3 oz)	150	100	9
Lean Cuisine Chicken Chow Mein With Rice	9 oz	240	300	6
HOME RECIPE				
chop suey w/ beef & pork	1 cup	300	600	33
chow mein, chicken	1 cup	255	280	10
MIX				
La Choy Dinner Classics Sweet & Sour	¾ cup	310	600	3
TAKE-OUT				
chicken teriyaki	¾ cup	399	443	tr
chop suey w/ pork	1 cup	375	215	58
chow mein, pork	1 cup	425	214	15
chow mein, shrimp	1 cup	221	236	15
fried rice	6.6 oz	249	0	2
fried rice w/ egg	6.7 oz	395	335	tr
wonton soup	1 cup	205	807	5
wonton, fried	½ cup (1 oz)	111	356	1

OYSTERS
(The vitamin A in prepared oyster dishes comes from animal sources.)

battered & fried	6 (4.9 oz)	368	363	4
breaded & fried	6 (4.9 oz)	368	363	4
stew	1 cup	278	892	4

FOOD	PORTION	CAL	VIT A	VIT C

PANCAKE/WAFFLE SYRUP

FOOD	PORTION	CAL	VIT A	VIT C
low calorie	1 tbsp	12	0	0
maple	2 tbsp	122	0	0

PANCAKES
(The vitamin in pancakes comes from animal ingredients like milk and egg.)

FROZEN

FOOD	PORTION	CAL	VIT A	VIT C
Blueberry (Aunt Jemima)	3.48 oz	220	110	0
Blueberry Microwave (Pillsbury)	3	250	0	1
Buttermilk (Aunt Jemima)	3.48 oz	210	0	0
Buttermilk Batter, as prep (Aunt Jemima)	3.6 oz	180	0	0
Buttermilk Microwave (Pillsbury)	3	260	0	0
Harvest Wheat Microwave (Pillsbury)	3	240	0	1
Lite Buttermilk (Aunt Jemima)	3.48 oz	140	0	0
Original (Aunt Jemima)	3.48 oz	211	69	0
Original Batter, as prep (Aunt Jemima)	3.6 oz	183	0	0
Original Microwave (Pillsbury)	3	240	0	0

HOME RECIPE

FOOD	PORTION	CAL	VIT A	VIT C
blueberry	1 (4-in diam)	84	76	1
plain	1 (4-in diam)	86	75	tr

MIX

FOOD	PORTION	CAL	VIT A	VIT C
Blueberry (Hungry Jack)	3 (4-in diam)	320	100	0
Buttermilk (Hungry Jack)	3 (4-in diam)	240	200	0
Buttermilk Complete (Hungry Jack)	3 (4-in diam)	180	0	0
Buttermilk Complete Packets (Hungry Jack)	3 (4-in diam)	180	0	0

FOOD	PORTION	CAL	VIT A	VIT C
Extra Lights (Hungry Jack)	3 (4-in diam)	210	200	0
Extra Lights Complete (Hungry Jack)	3 (4-in diam)	190	0	0
Pancake Mix, not prep (Health Valley)	1 oz	100	3	1
Panshakes (Hungry Jack)	3 (4-in diam)	250	100	0
buckwheat	1 (4-in diam)	62	70	tr
sugar free, low sodium	1 (3-in diam)	44	14	0
whole wheat	1 (4-in diam)	92	99	tr
TAKE-OUT buckwheat	1 (4-in diam)	55	60	tr
potato	1 (4-in diam)	78	27	4
w/ butter & syrup	3	519	281	3

PAPAYA

FRESH cubed	1 cup	54	2819	87
papaya	1	117	6122	188
JUICE Goya Nectar	6 oz	110	400	15
Kern's Nectar	6 oz	110	750	27
Libby's Nectar	6 oz	110	750	12
nectar	1 cup	142	277	8

PAPRIKA

paprika	1 tsp	6	1273	1

PARSLEY

Dole, chopped	1 tbsp	10	520	9
dry	1 tbsp	1	253	1
dry	1 tsp	1	70	tr
fresh, chopped	½ cup	11	1560	40

FOOD	PORTION	CAL	VIT A	VIT C

PARSNIPS

FRESH

cooked	1 (5.6 oz)	130	0	21
cooked, sliced	½ cup	63	0	10
raw, sliced	½ cup	50	0	11

PASSION FRUIT

purple	1	18	126	5

JUICE

purple	1 cup	126	1771	74
yellow	1 cup	149	5953	45

PASTA
(The vitamin A in pasta comes from animal sources like egg or from plant sources like spinach.)

DRY

Egg (Prince)	2 oz	221	130	0
Lasagna Spinach Whole Wheat (Health Valley)	2 oz	170	2869	4
Lasagna Whole Wheat (Health Valley)	2 oz	170	5	3
Pasta (Golden Grain)	2 oz	203	0	0
Rainbow (Prince)	2 oz	210	0	0
Spaghetti, Amaranth (Health Valley)	2 oz	170	0	2
Spaghetti, Spinach Whole Wheat (Health Valley)	2 oz	170	2869	4
Spaghetti, Oat Bran (Health Valley)	2 oz	120	9	1
Spaghetti, Whole Wheat (Health Valley)	2 oz	170	5	3
Spinach, Egg (Prince)	2 oz	220	0	0
corn, cooked	1 cup	176	80	0
elbows	1 cup	389	0	0

FOOD	PORTION	CAL	VIT A	VIT C
elbows, cooked	1 cup	197	0	0
shells	1 cup	389	0	0
shells, cooked	1 cup	197	0	0
spaghetti	2 oz	211	0	0
spirals	1 cup	389	0	0
spirals, cooked	1 cup	197	0	0
vegetable	1 cup	308	134	0
vegetable, cooked	1 cup	171	71	0
HOME RECIPE				
Made w/ egg, cooked	2 oz	74	33	0
made w/o egg, cooked	2 oz	71	0	0

PASTA DINNERS
(The vitamin A in pasta dinners comes from both animal and plant sources.)

FOOD	PORTION	CAL	VIT A	VIT C
Chef Boyardee Lasagna In Garden Vegetable Sauce	7.5 oz	170	750	2
Chef Boyardee Microwave Main Meal				
Beans & Pasta	10.5 oz	200	300	1
Ravioli Suprema	10.5 oz	290	750	4
Cheese Ravioli Suprema	10.5 oz	290	500	4
Fettuccine	10.5 oz	290	750	6
Lasagna	10.5 oz	290	500	4
Meat Tortellini	10.5 oz	220	500	6
Peas & Pasta	10.5 oz	190	750	4
Spaghetti Suprema	10.5 oz	200	500	2
Ziti In Sauce	10.5 oz	210	750	4
Chef Boyardee				
Pasta Rings & Meatballs	7.5 oz	220	400	1
Rigatoni	7.5 oz	210	500	5

FOOD	PORTION	CAL	VIT A	VIT C
Rings & Franks	7.5 oz	190	300	4
Shells In Meat Sauce	7.5 oz	210	500	5
Shells In Mushroom Sauce	7.5 oz	170	500	4
Turtles In Sauce	7.5 oz	160	200	1
Turtles w/ Meatballs	7.5 oz	210	300	1
Franco-American				
Beef RavioliO's In Meat Sauce	½ can (7½ oz)	250	500	6
CircusO's Pasta With Meatballs In Tomato Sauce	½ can (7⅜ oz)	210	500	4
SportyO's Pasta With Meatballs In Tomato Sauce	½ can (7⅜ oz)	210	500	4
TeddyO's Pasta With Meatballs	½ can (7⅜ oz)	210	500	4
Healthy Choice				
Lasagne With Meat Sauce	½ can (7.5 oz)	220	1500	5
Spaghetti Rings	½ can (7.5 oz)	140	500	2
Spaghetti With Meat Sauce	½ can (7.5 oz)	150	500	5
DRY MIX				
Kraft Mild American Style Spaghetti Dinner	1 cup	300	1000	6
Kraft Spaghetti With Meat Sauce Dinner	1 cup	360	500	2
Kraft Tangy Italian Style Spaghetti Dinner	1 cup	310	1000	9
Lipton Pasta And Sauce Cheddar Broccoli	½ cup	132	97	1
Lipton Pasta And Sauce Creamy Garlic	½ cup	146	73	0
Lipton Pasta And Sauce Creamy Mushroom	½ cup	143	420	1
Lipton Pasta And Sauce Herb Tomato	½ cup	130	456	1

FOOD	PORTION	CAL	VIT A	VIT C
Minute Microwave Cheddar Cheese Broccoli And Pasta, as prep	½ cup	160	200	2
Ultra Slim-Fast Macaroni & Cheese	2.3 oz	230	750	18
FROZEN				
Banquet Macaroni & Cheese	9 oz	240	100	9
Birds Eye Easy Recipe Chicken Primavera, not prep	½ pkg	80	2500	36
Birds Eye Easy Recipe Chicken Alfredo, not prep	½ pkg	160	750	15
Budget Gourmet				
Cheese Lasagna With Vegetables	1 pkg	290	4000	5
Cheese Manicotti	1 pkg	430	5000	6
Cheese Ravioli	1 pkg	290	400	4
Cheese Tortellini	1 pkg	210	4500	5
Italian Sausage Lasagna	1 pkg	430	5000	12
Lasagne With Meat Sauce	1 pkg	300	6000	9
Linguini With Scallops And Clams	1 pkg	290	750	9
Linguini With Shrimp And Clams	1 pkg	270	5000	6
Macaroni & Cheese	1 pkg	240	600	1
Pasta Alfredo With Broccoli	1 pkg	230	400	5
Shrimp With Fettucini	1 pkg	370	750	2
Three Cheese Lasagne	1 pkg	390	5000	9
Ziti In Marinara Sauce	1 pkg	200	2500	5
Dining Light				
Cheese Cannelloni	9 oz	310	750	5
Cheese Lasagna	9 oz	260	2000	6
Fettucini	9 oz	290	300	21
Lasagne	9 oz	240	1250	6
Spaghetti	9 oz	220	1000	12

FOOD	PORTION	CAL	VIT A	VIT C
Green Giant				
Garden Gourmet Creamy Mushroom	1 pkg	220	750	1
Garden Gourmet Pasta Dijon	1 pkg	260	1250	30
Garden Gourmet Pasta Florentine	1 pkg	230	9500	2
Garden Gourmet Rotini Cheddar	1 pkg	230	11000	30
One Serve Cheese Tortellini	1 pkg	260	1250	5
One Serve Macaroni And Cheese	1 pkg	230	300	0
One Serve Pasta Marinara	1 pkg	180	1250	6
One Serve Pasta Parmesan With Green Peas	1 pkg	170	200	5
Pasta Accents Creamy Cheddar	½ cup	100	3500	15
Pasta Accents Garden Herb	½ cup	80	3000	15
Pasta Accents Garlic Seasoning	½ cup	110	2250	15
Pasta Accents Pasta Primavera	½ cup	110	400	15
Healthy Choice				
Baked Cheese Ravioli	9 oz	240	2500	5
Cheese Manicotti	9.25 oz	230	1250	6
Lasagna With Meat Sauce	10 oz	260	750	2
Linguini With Shrimp	9.5 oz	230	500	12
Pasta Primavera	11 oz	280	3500	30
Pasta With Shrimp	12.5 oz	270	500	9
Rigatoni In Meat Sauce	9.5 oz	240	1750	5
Rigatoni With Chicken	12.5 oz	360	300	9
Spaghetti With Meat Sauce	10 oz	280	1250	5
Teriyaki Pasta With Chicken	12.6 oz	350	500	6
Zucchini Lasagna	11.5 oz	240	1750	6

FOOD	PORTION	CAL	VIT A	VIT C
Kid Cuisine				
Macaroni & Cheese With Mini Franks	9 oz	360	100	4
Mini-Cheese Ravioli	8.75 oz	290	1250	1
Spaghetti With Meat Sauce	9.25 oz	310	1250	2
Le Menu				
LightStyle 3-Cheese Stuffed Shells	10 oz	280	1250	30
LightStyle Cheese Tortellini	10 oz	230	4200	42
Manicotti With Three Cheeses	11¾ oz	390	1000	15
Le Menu Entree LightStyle				
Lasagna With Meat Sauce	10 oz	290	1250	18
Meat Sauce & Cheese Tortellini	8 oz	250	500	42
Spaghetti With Beef Sauce And Mushrooms	9 oz	280	750	36
Garden Vegetables Lasagna	10½ oz	260	1250	48
Lean Cuisine				
Beef Cannelloni With Mornay Sauce	9.6 oz	210	1000	6
Cheese Cannelloni With Tomato Sauce	9.1 oz	270	300	21
Cheese Ravioli	8.5 oz	240	300	36
Lasagne With Meat Sauce	10¼ oz	260	500	6
Macaroni And Beef In Tomato Sauce	10 oz	240	500	1
Rigatoni Bake With Meat Sauce And Cheese	9¾ oz	250	1000	6
Spaghetti And Meatballs	9½ oz	280	300	4
Spaghetti With Meat Sauce	11.5 oz	290	500	6
Tuna Lasagna With Spinach Noodles And Vegetables	9.75 oz	240	2250	4
Zucchini Lasagna	11 oz	260	1750	12

FOOD	PORTION	CAL	VIT A	VIT C
Morton Spaghetti & Meat Sauce	8.5 oz	170	3000	9
Mrs. Paul's Light Seafood Entree Seafood Lasagne	9½ oz	290	100	2
Mrs. Paul's Seafood Rotini	9 oz	240	tr	1
Swanson				
Homestyle Lasagne With Meat Sauce	10½ oz	400	750	6
Homestyle Macaroni & Cheese	10 oz	390	100	1
Homestyle Spaghetti With Itallan Style Meatballs	13 oz	490	1250	12
Macaroni & Cheese	12¼ oz	370	3500	6
Spaghetti & Meatballs	12½ oz	390	750	12
Ultra Slim-Fast Pasta Primavera	12 oz	340	4000	15
Ultra Slim-Fast Spaghetti With Beef & Mushroom Sauce	12 oz	370	500	5
HOME RECIPE				
macaroni & cheese	1 cup	430	860	1
spaghetti w/ meatballs & tomato sauce	1 cup	330	1590	22
SHELF STABLE				
Healthy Choice				
Lasagne w/ Meat Sauce	7.5 oz cup	220	1500	5
Spaghetti Rings	7.5 oz cup	140	500	2
Spaghetti w/ Meat Sauce	7.5 oz cup	150	500	5
TAKE-OUT				
lasagna	1 piece (2.5 × 2.5 in)	374	1315	13
lasagne	8 oz	347	1815	tr
macaroni & cheese	1 cup	230	260	tr
manicotti	¾ cup (6.4 oz)	273	2613	12
rigatoni w/ sausage sauce	¾ cup	260	999	16

FOOD	PORTION	CAL	VIT A	VIT C
spaghetti w/ meatballs & cheese	1 cup	407	2724	45

PASTA SALAD
(The vitamin A in pasta salad comes from both animal ingredients like mayonnaise and plant sources like vegetables.)

MIX
Kraft Pasta Salad And Dressing

Broccoli And Vegetables	½ cup	210	400	2
Garden Primavera	½ cup	170	450	1
Light Italian	½ cup	130	200	1
Lipton Robust Italian	½ cup	126	390	1

TAKE-OUT

italian style pasta salad	3.5 oz	140	300	9

PÂTÉ
(The vitamin A in pâté comes from animal sources.)

CANNED

liver	1 oz	90	936	0
liver	1 tbsp (13 g)	41	429	0

PEACH

Clingstone Halves (S&W)	½ cup	100	500	2
Clingstone Halves Unsweetened (S&W)	½ cup	30	500	4
Clingstone Halves Diet (S&W)	½ cup	30	500	4
Clingstone Sliced Unsweetened (S&W)	½ cup	30	500	4
Clingstone Sliced Diet (S&W)	½ cup	30	500	4
Freestone Halves Diet (S&W)	½ cup	30	200	1
Freestone Halves in Heavy Syrup (S&W)	½ cup	100	250	1
Freestone Sliced in Heavy Syrup (S&W)	½ cup	100	200	1

FOOD	PORTION	CAL	VIT A	VIT C
Freestone Slices Diet (S&W)	½ cup	30	200	1
Halves (Hunt's)	4 oz	90	40	3
Sliced Yellow Cling Natural Style (S&W)	½ cup	90	500	6
Slices (Hunt's)	4 oz	90	40	3
Yellow Cling Natural Lite (S&W)	½ cup	50	50	9
Yellow Cling Sliced Premium in Heavy Syrup (S&W)	½ cup	100	500	2
Yellow Cling Whole Spiced in Heavy Syrup (S&W)	½ cup	90	750	2
halves in heavy syrup	1 half	60	269	2
halves in juice pack	1 half	34	294	3
halves in light syrup	1 half	44	286	2
halves water pack	1 half	18	410	2
spiced in heavy syrup	1 cup	180	768	13
spiced in heavy syrup	1 fruit	66	279	5
DRIED				
halves	1 cup	383	3461	8
halves	10	311	2812	6
halves, cooked w/ sugar	½ cup	139	243	5
halves, cooked w/o sugar	½ cup	99	254	5
FRESH				
peach	1	37	465	6
sliced	1 cup	73	910	11
FROZEN				
slices, sweetened	1 cup	235	709	235
JUICE				
Dole Pure & Light	6 oz	100	26	1
Goya Nectar	6 oz	110	414	1
Libby's Ripe Nectar	8 oz	130	500	21
Smucker's	8 oz	120	500	6
Nectar	1 cup	134	643	13

FOOD	PORTION	CAL	VIT A	VIT C
PEANUT BUTTER				
Health Valley Chunky No Salt	2 tbsp	170	0	tr
Health Valley Creamy No Salt	2 tbsp	170	0	tr
Smucker's				
Goober Grape	2 tbsp	180	0	0
Honey Sweetened	2 tbsp	200	0	0
Natural	2 tbsp	200	0	0
Natural No-Salt Added	2 tbsp	200	0	0
chunky	1 cup	1520	0	0
chunky	2 tbsp	188	0	0
chunky w/o salt	1 cup	1520	0	0
chunky w/o salt	2 tbsp	188	0	0
smooth	1 cup	1517	0	0
smooth	2 tbsp	188	0	0
smooth w/o salt	1 cup	1517	0	0
smooth w/o salt	2 tbsp	188	0	0
PEANUTS				
cooked	½ cup	102	0	0
dry roasted	1 cup	855	0	0
dry roasted	1 oz	164	0	0
oil roasted	1 cup	837	0	0
oil roasted	1 oz	163	0	0
oil roasted w/o salt	1 cup	837	0	0
oil roasted w/o salt	1 oz	163	0	0
spanish oil roasted	1 oz	162	0	0
spanish oil roasted w/o salt	1 oz	162	0	0
unroasted	1 oz	159	0	0
valencia oil roasted	1 cup	848	0	0
valencia oil roasted	1 oz	165	0	0

FOOD	PORTION	CAL	VIT A	VIT C
valencia oil roasted w/o salt	1 cup	848	0	0
valencia oil roasted w/o salt	1 oz	165	0	0
virginia oil roasted	1 cup	826	0	0
virginia oil roasted	1 oz	161	0	0

PEAR

CANNED
Halves (Hunt's)	4 oz	90	0	1
halves in heavy syrup	1 cup	188	0	3
halves in heavy syrup	1 half	68	0	1
halves in juice pack	1 cup	123	14	4
halves in light syrup	1 half	45	0	1
halves in water pack	1 half	22	0	1

DRIED
halves	1 cup	472	6	13
halves	10	459	6	12
halves, cooked w/ sugar	½ cup	196	56	5
halves, cooked w/o sugar	½ cup	163	54	5

FRESH
asian	1 (4.3 oz)	51	0	2
pear	1	98	33	7
sliced w/ skin	1 cup	97	33	7

JUICE
Goya Nectar	6 oz	120	<100	19
nectar	1 cup	149	1	3

PEAS

CANNED
Field Peas (Trappey's)	½ cup	90	tr	tr
Field Peas With Snaps (Trappey's)	½ cup	90	tr	tr
Petit Pois (S&W)	½ cup	70	400	12

FOOD	PORTION	CAL	VIT A	VIT C
Sweet (Green Giant)	½ cup	50	300	6
Sweet (S&W)	½ cup	70	400	12
Sweet Water Pack (S&W)	½ cup	40	300	11
Veri-Green Sweet (S&W)	½ cup	70	400	12
green	½ cup	59	653	8
green, low sodium	½ cup	59	653	8
DRIED				
split, cooked	1 cup	231	14	1
FRESH				
Dole Sugar Peas	½ cup	30	105	43
edible-pod, cooked	½ cup	34	104	38
edible-pod, raw	½ cup	30	105	43
green, cooked	½ cup	67	478	11
green, raw	½ cup	58	461	29
FROZEN				
Big Valley	3.3 oz	80	750	18
Chinese Pea Pods (Chun King)	1.5 oz	20	100	9
Green (Birds Eye)	½ cup	80	750	18
Harvest Fresh Early June (Green Giant)	½ cup	60	500	15
Harvest Fresh Sugar Snap (Green Giant)	½ cup	30	200	6
Harvest Fresh Sweet (Green Giant)	½ cup	50	300	6
In Butter Sauce (Birds Eye)	½ cup	80	500	15
In Butter Sauce (Green Giant)	½ cup	80	500	9
Le Suer Early Select (Green Giant)	½ cup	60	500	12
Le Suer Early In Butter Sauce (Green Giant)	½ cup	80	500	9
One Serve In Butter Sauce (Green Giant)	1 pkg	90	500	12

FOOD	PORTION	CAL	VIT A	VIT C
Polybag Deluxe Tender Tiny (Birds Eye)	½ cup	60	750	18
Polybag Green (Birds Eye)	½ cup	70	750	18
Snow Pea Pods (Le Choy)	½ pkg (3 oz)	35	200	18
Sugar Snap Deluxe (Birds Eye)	½ cup	45	400	21
Sugar Snap Sweet Select (Green Giant)	½ cup	30	200	9
Sweet (Green Giant)	½ cup	50	300	9
Tender Tiny Deluxe (Birds Eye)	½ cup	60	750	18
edible-pod, cooked	1 pkg (10 oz)	132	421	56
edible-pod, cooked	½ cup	42	133	18
green, cooked	½ cup	63	534	8
SPROUTS raw	½ cup	77	100	6
TAKE-OUT pea & potato curry	1 serving (7 oz)	284	550	12
pea curry	1 serving (4.4 oz)	438	2600	14

PECANS

FOOD	PORTION	CAL	VIT A	VIT C
dried	1 oz	190	36	1
halves, dried	1 cup	721	138	2

PEPPER

FOOD	PORTION	CAL	VIT A	VIT C
cayenne	1 tsp	6	749	1
red	1 tsp	6	749	1

PEPPERS

FOOD	PORTION	CAL	VIT A	VIT C
CANNED Hot Cherry (Vlasic)	1 oz	10	100	15
Mild Cherry (Vlasic)	1 oz	8	100	6
chili, green hot	1 (2.6 oz)	18	445	50

FOOD	PORTION	CAL	VIT A	VIT C
chili, green hot, chopped	½ cup	17	415	46
chili, red hot	1 (2.6 oz)	18	8681	50
chili, red hot, chopped	½ cup	17	8087	46
green halves	½ cup	13	109	33
jalapeno, chopped	½ cup	17	1156	9
red halves	½ cup	13	364	33
DRIED				
green	1 tbsp	1	25	8
red	1 tbsp	1	309	8
FRESH				
Dole Bell	1 med	25	415	117
chili, green, hot, raw	1	18	346	109
chili, green, hot, raw, chopped	½ cup	30	578	182
chili, red, hot, raw	1 (1.6 oz)	18	4838	109
chili, red, raw, chopped	½ cup	30	8063	182
green, chopped, cooked	½ cup	19	403	51
green, cooked	1 (2.6 oz)	20	432	54
green, raw	1 (2.6 oz)	20	468	95
green, raw, chopped	½ cup	13	316	45
red, chopped, cooked	½ cup	19	2745	125
red, cooked	1 (2.6 oz)	20	2745	125
red, raw	1 (2.6 oz)	20	4218	141
red, raw, chopped	½ cup	13	2850	95
yellow, raw	1 (6.5 oz)	50	442	341
yellow, raw	10 strips	14	124	95
FROZEN				
green, chopped, not prep	1 oz	6	103	16
red, chopped	1 oz	6	1333	16

FOOD	PORTION	CAL	VIT A	VIT C

PERCH
(The vitamin A in perch comes from animal sources.)

FRESH
red, raw	3½ oz	114	tr	1

PERSIMMONS

dried japanese	1	93	190	0
fresh japanese	1	118	3640	13

PHEASANT
(The vitamin A in pheasant comes from animal sources.)

FRESH
breast w/o skin, raw	½ breast (6.4 oz)	243	268	11
w/ skin, raw	½ pheasant (14 oz)	723	706	21
w/o skin, raw	½ pheasant (12.4 oz)	470	181	21

PHYLLO DOUGH
(The vitamin A in phyllo dough comes from animal ingredients like butter.)

Ekizian	½ lb	865	520	0
phyllo dough	1 oz	85	0	0
sheet	1	57	0	0

PICKLES

Hot & Spicy Garden Mix (Vlasic)	1 oz	4	100	4
dill	1 (2.3 oz)	12	214	1
dill, low sodium	1 (2.3 oz)	12	214	1
dill, low sodium, sliced	1 slice	1	20	tr
dill, sliced	1 slice	1	20	tr
gherkins	3½ oz	21	0	2

FOOD	PORTION	CAL	VIT A	VIT C
kosher dill	1 (2.3 oz)	12	214	1
polish dill	1 (2.3 oz)	12	214	1
quick sour	1 (1.2 oz)	4	51	tr
quick sour, low sodium	1 (1.2 oz)	4	51	tr
quick sour, sliced	1 slice	1	10	tr
sweet	1 (1.2 oz)	41	44	tr
sweet gherkin	1 sm (½ oz)	20	10	1
sweet, low sodium	1 (1.2 oz)	41	44	tr
sweet, sliced	1 slice	7	8	tr

PIE
(The vitamin A in pie comes from animal ingredients; the exceptions are peach and pumpkin rich in plant sources.)

FOOD	PORTION	CAL	VIT A	VIT C
CANNED FILLING				
pumpkin pie mix	1 cup	282	22405	10
FROZEN				
Apple Streusel Free & Light (Sara Lee)	1 slice (2.9 oz)	170	100	1
Cherry (Banquet)	1 slice (3.3 oz)	250	100	1
Peach (Banquet)	1 slice (3.3 oz)	245	200	12
Peach Homestyle (Sara Lee)	1 slice (3.4 oz)	280	100	12
Pumpkin (Banquet)	1 slice (3.3 oz)	200	1750	1
HOME RECIPE				
pecan	⅙ pie 9 in	575	220	0
MIX				
Banana Cream, as prep w/ whole milk	⅙ pie (8 in)	103	102	1
Jell-O				
Chocolate Mousse	⅛ pie	259	393	1
Coconut Cream	⅛ pie	258	381	1
Coconut Cream, as prep w/ whole milk	⅙ pie (8 in)	111	102	1
Pumpkin	⅛ pie	253	386	1

FOOD	PORTION	CAL	VIT A	VIT C
READY-TO-USE				
apple	⅙ pie (9 in)	405	50	2
blueberry	⅙ pie (9 in)	380	140	6
cherry	⅙ pie (9 in)	410	700	0
creme	⅙ pie (9 in)	455	210	0
custard	⅙ pie (9 in)	330	350	0
lemon meringue	⅙ pie (9 in)	355	240	4
peach	⅙ pie (9 in)	405	1150	5
pumpkin	⅙ pie (9 in)	320	3750	0
SNACK				
Apple (Drake's)	1 (2 oz)	210	tr	tr
Blueberry (Drake's)	1 (2 oz)	210	tr	tr
Cherry (Drake's)	1 (2 oz)	220	tr	tr
Lemon (Drake's)	1 (2 oz)	210	tr	tr
apple	1 (3 oz)	266	148	1
cherry	1 (3 oz)	266	148	1
lemon	1 (3 oz)	266	148	1

PIE CRUST

FOOD	PORTION	CAL	VIT A	VIT C
FROZEN				
puff pastry, baked	1 shell (1.4 oz)	223	0	0
HOME RECIPE				
9-inch crust	1	900	0	0
MIX				
Pillsbury Stick	⅙ of a 2-crust pie	270	0	0
Pillsbury Mix	⅙ of 2-crust pie	270	0	0
Pillsbury Mix, as prep	2 crusts	1485	0	0
REFRIGERATED				
Pillsbury All Ready	⅛ of 2-crust pie	240	0	0

FOOD	PORTION	CAL	VIT A	VIT C

PIEROGI
TAKE-OUT

pierogi	¾ cup (4.4 oz)	307	246	1

PIG'S EARS AND FEET

ears, frzn, simmered	1 ear (3.7 oz)	183	0	0
feet, pickled	1 lb	923	0	0
feet, pickled	1 oz	58	0	0
feet, simmered	2.5 oz	138	0	0

PIGEON PEAS
DRIED

cooked	1 cup	204	4	0
cooked	½ cup	102	2	0

PIKE
FRESH
(The vitamin A in pike comes from plant sources.)

northern, cooked	½ fillet (5.4 oz)	176	125	6
northern, raw	3 oz	75	60	3

PIMIENTOS

Dromedary	1 oz	10	500	9
canned	1 slice	0	27	1
canned	1 tbsp	3	319	10

PINE NUTS

pinyon dried	1 oz	161	8	1

PINEAPPLE
CANNED

All Cuts Juice Pack (Dole)	½ cup	70	50	4
All Cuts Syrup Pack (Dole)	½ cup	90	65	4

FOOD	PORTION	CAL	VIT A	VIT C
chunks in heavy syrup	1 cup	199	37	19
chunks in juice pack	1 cup	150	95	24
crushed in heavy syrup	1 cup	199	37	19
slices in heavy syrup	1 slice	45	8	4
slices in juice pack	1 slice	35	22	6
slices in light syrup	1 slice	30	9	4
slices in water pack	1 slice	19	9	5
tidbits in heavy syrup	1 cup	199	37	19
tidbits in juice	1 cup	150	95	24
tidbits in water	1 cup	79	37	19
FRESH				
Dole	2 slices	90	46	16
diced	1 cup	77	35	24
slice	1 slice	42	19	13
FROZEN				
chunks, sweetened	½ cup	104	37	10
JUICE				
Dole New Breakfast Juice	6 oz	100	1058	60
canned	1 cup	139	12	27
frzn, as prep	1 cup	129	25	30
frzn, not prep	6 oz	387	108	91

PINK BEANS

FOOD	PORTION	CAL	VIT A	VIT C
CANNED				
Goya Spanish Style	7.5 oz	140	1140	2
DRIED				
cooked	1 cup	252	0	0

PINTO BEANS

FOOD	PORTION	CAL	VIT A	VIT C
CANNED				
Goya Spanish Style	7.5 oz	140	1160	2
Green Giant	½ cup	90	0	0

FOOD	PORTION	CAL	VIT A	VIT C
Green Giant Picante	½ cup	100	300	0
Trappey's	½ cup	90	tr	tr
Trappey's Hearty Texas	½ cup	110	200	tr
Trappey's Jalapinto	½ cup	90	tr	tr
pinto	1 cup	186	3	2
DRIED				
cooked	1 cup	235	3	4
FROZEN				
cooked	3 oz	152	0	1

PITANGA

fresh	1	2	105	2
fresh	1 cup	57	2595	46

PIZZA

(The vitamin A in pizza comes from animal sources like cheese and meat and from plant sources like tomato sauce and vegetables.)

FOOD	PORTION	CAL	VIT A	VIT C
FROZEN				
Fox Deluxe				
Golden Topping	½ pizza	240	200	1
Hamburger	½ pizza	260	100	1
Pepperoni	½ pizza	250	100	1
Sausage	½ pizza	260	100	1
Sausage & Pepperoni	½ pizza	260	100	1
Healthy Choice French Bread				
Cheese	1 (5.3 oz)	270	200	5
Deluxe	1 (6.25 oz)	330	300	12
Italian Turkey Sausage	1 (6.45 oz)	320	300	15
Pepperoni	1 (6.25 oz)	320	400	21
Jeno's				
4-Pack Cheese	1 pizza	160	200	1
4-Pack Combination	1 pizza	180	100	1
4-Pack Hamburger	1 pizza	180	100	1

FOOD	PORTION	CAL	VIT A	VIT C
4-Pack Pepperoni	1 pizza	170	100	1
4-Pack Sausage	1 pizza	180	100	1
Crisp 'n Tasty Canadian Bacon	½ pizza	250	200	5
Crisp 'n Tasty Cheese	½ pizza	270	400	2
Crisp 'n Tasty Hamburger	½ pizza	290	200	2
Crisp 'n Tasty Pepperoni	½ pizza	280	200	2
Crisp 'n Tasty Sausage	½ pizza	300	200	2
Crisp 'n Tasty Sausage & Pepperoni	½ pizza	300	200	2
Microwave Pizza Rolls Pepperoni & Cheese	6	240	300	6
Microwave Pizza Rolls Sausage & Cheese	6	250	200	6
Pizza Rolls Cheese	6	240	300	1
Pizza Rolls Hamburger	6	240	100	0
Pizza Rolls Pepperoni & Cheese	6	230	200	6
Pizza Rolls Sausage & Pepperoni	6	230	100	4
Kid Cuisine Cheese	1 (6.85 oz)	380	1250	4
Kid Cuisine Hamburger	1 (6.85 oz)	330	200	4
MicroMagic Deep Dish Combination	1 (6.5 oz)	605	1250	5
Pepperoni	1 (6.5 oz)	615	1750	5
Sausage	1 (6.5 oz)	590	500	5
Mr. P's Combination	½ pizza	260	100	1
Golden Topping	½ pizza	240	200	1
Hamburger	½ pizza	260	100	1
Pepperoni	½ pizza	250	100	1
Sausage	½ pizza	260	100	1

FOOD	PORTION	CAL	VIT A	VIT C
Pappalo's French Bread				
Cheese	1 pizza	360	500	5
Combination	1 pizza	430	500	6
Pepperoni	1 pizza	410	500	5
Sausage	1 pizza	410	500	5
Pappalo's Thin Crust				
Combination	⅙ pizza	260	400	4
Hamburger	⅙ pizza	240	400	4
Pepperoni	⅙ pizza	270	500	4
Sausage	⅙ pizza	250	400	4
Pappalo's Pan				
Combination	⅙ pizza	340	500	2
Hamburger	⅙ pizza	310	500	2
Pepperoni	⅙ pizza	330	500	2
Sausage	⅙ pizza	360	400	2
Pepperidge Farm Croissant Pastry				
Cheese	1	430	300	2
Deluxe	1	440	200	1
Pepperoni	1	420	300	4
Pillsbury Microwave				
Cheese	½ pizza	240	400	4
Combination	½ pizza	310	400	9
French Bread	1 pizza	370	100	1
French Bread Pepperoni	1 pizza	430	200	0
French Bread Sausage	1 pizza	410	200	0
French Bread Sausage & Pepperoni	1 pizza	450	200	2
Pepperoni	½ pizza	300	400	9
Sausage	½ pizza	280	400	9
Totino's				
Microwave Cheese	1 pizza	250	100	0

FOOD	PORTION	CAL	VIT A	VIT C
Microwave Pepperoni	1 pizza	280	500	5
Microwave Sausage	1 pizza	320	500	5
Microwave Sausage Pepperoni Combination	1 pizza	310	500	5
My Classic Deluxe Cheese	⅙ pizza	210	300	4
My Classic Deluxe Combination	⅙ pizza	270	300	4
My Classic Deluxe Pepperoni	⅙ pizza	260	300	4
Pan Pepperoni	⅙ pizza	330	400	2
Pan Sausage	¼ pizza	320	400	2
Pan Sausage & Pepperoni Combination	⅙ pizza	340	400	2
Pan Three Cheese	⅙ pizza	290	500	2
Party Bacon	½ pizza	370	400	4
Party Canadian Bacon	½ pizza	310	300	4
Party Cheese	½ pizza	340	500	4
Party Combination	½ pizza	380	400	4
Party Hamburger	½ pizza	370	300	4
Party Mexican Style	½ pizza	380	400	9
Party Pepperoni	½ pizza	370	400	4
Party Sausage	½ pizza	390	300	4
Party Vegetable	½ pizza	300	500	12
Slices Cheese	1	170	200	2
Slices Combination	1	200	200	2
Slices Pepperoni	1	190	300	2
Slices Sausage	1	200	200	2
SAUCES				
Ragu Pizza Quick Sauce				
Garlic & Basil	1.7 fl oz	35	300	4
Mushrooms	1.7 fl oz	35	300	4
Traditional	1.7 fl oz	35	300	4

FOOD	PORTION	CAL	VIT A	VIT C
Ragu Pizza Quick Sauce *(cont.)*				
w/ Cheese	1.7 fl oz	35	300	4
w/ Pepperoni	1.7 fl oz	35	300	4
w/ Sausage	3 tbsp	35	300	4
TAKE-OUT				
cheese	⅛ pie (12 in)	140	382	1
cheese	12-in pie	1121	3051	10
cheese, meat & vegetables	⅛ pie (12 in)	184	524	2
cheese, meat & vegetables	12-in pie	1472	4184	13
pepperoni	⅛ pie (12 in)	181	282	2
pepperoni	12-in pie	1445	2250	13

PLANTAINS

FOOD	PORTION	CAL	VIT A	VIT C
FRESH				
sliced, cooked	½ cup	89	700	8
uncooked	1 (6.3 oz)	218	2017	33
TAKE-OUT				
ripe, fried	2.8 oz	214	80	10

PLUMS

FOOD	PORTION	CAL	VIT A	VIT C
CANNED				
Halves Unpeeled Diet (S&W)	½ cup	52	1250	2
Whole Unpeeled Diet (S&W)	½ cup	52	1250	2
purple in heavy syrup	1 cup	320	668	1
purple in heavy syrup	3	119	344	1
purple in juice pack	1 cup	146	2542	7
purple in juice pack	3	55	958	3
purple in light syrup	1 cup	158	666	1
purple in light syrup	3	83	352	1
purple in water pack	1 cup	102	2276	8
purple in water pack	3	39	868	3

FOOD	PORTION	CAL	VIT A	VIT C
FRESH				
plum	1	36	213	6
sliced	1 cup	91	533	16
JUICE				
Kern's Nectar	6 oz	110	300	27

POI

poi	½ cup	134	24	5

POKEBERRY SHOOTS

FOOD	PORTION	CAL	VIT A	VIT C
FRESH				
cooked	½ cup	16	7134	67
raw	½ cup	18	6960	109

POLLACK
(The vitamin A in pollack comes from animal sources.)

FROZEN				
Mrs. Paul's Light Fillets	1 fillet (4.5 oz)	240	tr	tr

POPCORN

FOOD	PORTION	CAL	VIT A	VIT C
Pillsbury Microwave				
Butter	3 cups	210	0	2
Original	3 cups	210	0	2
Salt Free	3 cups	170	0	2
Ultra Slim-Fast Lite N' Tasty	½ oz	60	500	6
air-popped	1 cup	30	10	0
popped w/ vegetable oil	1 cup	55	20	0
sugar syrup coated	1 cup	135	30	0

PORK
(The vitamin A in pork comes from animal sources.)

FOOD	PORTION	CAL	VIT A	VIT C
FRESH				
blade chop, roasted	1 (3.1 oz)	321	8	tr
center loin chop, broiled	1 (3.1 oz)	275	8	tr

FOOD	PORTION	CAL	VIT A	VIT C
center loin, roasted	3 oz	259	7	tr
loin w/ fat, roasted	3 oz	271	7	tr
shoulder blade roll, cured, lean & fat	3 oz	304	0	tr
shoulder whole, roasted	3 oz	277	7	tr
spleen, braised	3 oz	127	0	10
tenderloin, lean only, roasted	3 oz	141	6	tr

POT PIE
(The vitamin A in pot pies comes from animal sources and plant sources.)

FOOD	PORTION	CAL	VIT A	VIT C
FROZEN				
Beef Hungry Man (Swanson)	16 oz	610	2250	4
Chicken Homestyle (Swanson)	8 oz	410	1500	2
Vegetable Pie w/ Beef (Banquet)	7 oz	510	500	1
HOME RECIPE				
beef, baked	⅓ of 9-in pie (7.4 oz)	515	4220	6
chicken	⅓ of 9-in pie (8.1 oz)	545	7220	5

POTATO
(The vitamin A in potatoes comes from plant sources and from animal ingredients like cheese and bacon.)

FOOD	PORTION	CAL	VIT A	VIT C
FRESH				
baked skin only	1 skin (2 oz)	115	0	8
baked w/ skin	1 (6.5 oz)	220	0	26
baked w/o skin	1 (5 oz)	145	0	20
boiled	½ cup	68	0	10
raw w/o skin	1 (3.9 oz)	88	0	22
FROZEN				
Baked Potato Broccoli And Cheddar (Lean Cuisine)	10.4 oz	290	400	48

FOOD	PORTION	CAL	VIT A	VIT C
Baked Potato w/ Broccoli & Cheese Sauce (Healthy Choice)	10 oz	240	100	15
Cheddared Potatoes (Budget Gourmet)	1 pkg	260	300	6
Cheddared Potatoes With Broccoli (Budget Gourmet)	1 pkg	150	500	15
Nacho Potatoes (Budget Gourmet)	1 pkg	200	200	6
One Serve Potatoes And Broccoli In Cheese Sauce (Green Giant)	1 pkg	130	1750	30
One Serve Potatoes Au Gratin (Green Giant)	1 pkg	200	200	6
Stuffed Potatoes w/ Cheddar Cheese (Oh Boy!)	1 (6 oz)	150	500	4
Stuffed Potatoes w/ Real Bacon (Oh Boy!)	1 (6 oz)	120	100	5
Stuffed Potatoes w/ Sour Cream & Chives (Oh Boy!)	1 (6 oz)	110	200	2
Three Cheese Potatoes (Budget Gourmet)	1 pkg	230	300	6
Topped Broccoli & Cheese (Ore Ida)	1 (5.63 oz)	160	300	18
Topped Vegetable Primavera (Ore Ida)	1 (6.13 oz)	160	750	15
Twice Baked Butter Flavor (Ore Ida)	1 (5 oz)	200	100	4
Twice Baked Cheddar Cheese (Ore Ida)	1 (5 oz)	210	200	5
potato puffs	½ cup	138	10	4
potato puffs, as prep	1	16	1	1
HOME RECIPE				
au gratin	½ cup	160	322	12
mashed	½ cup	111	177	6

FOOD	PORTION	CAL	VIT A	VIT C
o'brien	1 cup	157	934	32
potato pancakes	1 (1.3 oz)	101	53	8
scalloped	½ cup	105	165	13
MIX				
Cheddar And Bacon Casserole (French's)	½ cup	130	100	1
Creamy Stroganoff (French's)	½ cup	130	100	4
Creamy Italian Scalloped (French's)	½ cup	120	100	1
Crispy Top Scalloped w/ Savory Onion (French's)	½ cup	140	100	1
Mashed Potato Flakes (Hungry Jack)	½ cup	40	300	5
Real Cheese Scalloped (French's)	½ cup	140	200	1
Real Sour Cream and Chives (French's)	½ cup	150	200	1
Spuds Mashed (French's)	½ cup	140	300	1
Tangy Au Gratin (French's)	½ cup	130	100	1
instant mashed flakes, as prep w/ whole milk & butter	½ cup	118	189	10
instant mashed granules, not prep	½ cup	372	9	37
instant mashed granules, as prep w/ whole milk & butter	½ cup	114	195	6
TAKE-OUT				
au gratin w/ cheese	½ cup	178	392	12
baked, topped w/ cheese sauce	1	475	834	26
baked, topped w/ cheese sauce & bacon	1	451	627	29
baked, topped w/ cheese sauce & broccoli	1	402	1695	49
baked, topped w/ cheese sauce & chili	1	481	768	32

FOOD	PORTION	CAL	VIT A	VIT C
baked, topped w/ sour cream & chives	1	394	1346	34
curry	1 serving (6 oz)	292	1000	14
french fried in beef tallow	1 lg	358	33	6
french fried in beef tallow	1 reg	237	22	4
french fried in vegetable oil	1 lg	355	33	6
french fried in vegetable oil	1 reg	235	22	4
hash browns	½ cup	151	18	6
mashed w/ whole milk & margarine	⅓ cup	66	33	tr
mustard potato salad	3.5 oz	120	500	12
potato salad	½ cup	179	261	13
potato salad	⅓ cup	108	95	1
scalloped	½ cup	127	196	13

PRETZELS

FOOD	PORTION	CAL	VIT A	VIT C
Ultra Slim-Fast Lite N' Tasty	1 oz	100	500	6
Wege Unsalted	1 oz	102	tr	tr
sticks	10	10	0	0
twist	1 (½ oz)	65	0	0
twists, thin	10 (2 oz)	240	0	0

PRICKLY PEAR

FOOD	PORTION	CAL	VIT A	VIT C
fresh	1	42	53	14

PRUNES

CANNED

FOOD	PORTION	CAL	VIT A	VIT C
in heavy syrup	1 cup	245	1866	7
in heavy syrup	5	90	686	2
DRIED				
cooked w/ sugar	½ cup	147	340	3

FOOD	PORTION	CAL	VIT A	VIT C
cooked w/o sugar	½ cup	113	324	3
dried	1 cup	385	3199	5
dried	10	201	1669	3
juice, canned	1 cup	181	9	11

PUDDING
(The vitamin A in pudding comes mostly from animal ingredients like milk, with a small amount coming from plant sources.)

FOOD	PORTION	CAL	VIT A	VIT C
HOME RECIPE				
bread w/ raisins	½ cup	180	125	1
corn	⅔ cup	181	411	5
yorkshire, as prep w/ skim milk	3.5 oz	93	75	1
yorkshire, as prep w/ whole milk	3.5 oz	104	165	1
MIX WITH 2% MILK				
Jell-O				
Banana Instant Sugar Free	½ cup	84	250	1
Chocolate Instant Sugar Free	½ cup	92	251	1
Chocolate Sugar Free	½ cup	91	252	1
Pistachio Instant Sugar Free	½ cup	94	250	1
Vanilla Instant Sugar Free	½ cup	82	250	1
MIX WITH SKIM MILK				
Butterscotch (D-Zerta)	½ cup	68	250	1
Chocolate (D-Zerta)	½ cup	65	251	1
Vanilla (D-Zerta)	½ cup	69	250	1
MIX WITH WHOLE MILK				
Jell-O				
Banana Cream Instant	½ cup	165	154	1
Butter Pecan Instant	½ cup	170	154	1
Butterscotch	½ cup	169	154	1

FOOD	PORTION	CAL	VIT A	VIT C
Butterscotch Instant	½ cup	164	154	1
Chocolate Instant	½ cup	176	155	1
Chocolate Tapioca Americana	½ cup	169	156	1
Chocolate Fudge Instant	½ cup	175	156	1
Coconut Cream Instant	½ cup	178	154	1
French Vanilla	½ cup	169	154	1
French Vanilla Instant	½ cup	165	154	1
Lemon Instant	½ cup	168	154	1
Milk Chocolate Instant	½ cup	179	161	1
Pineapple Cream Instant	½ cup	165	154	1
Pistachio Instant	½ cup	170	154	1
Rice Americana	½ cup	175	154	1
Vanilla	½ cup	156	154	1
Vanilla Instant	½ cup	168	154	1
Vanilla Tapioca Americana	½ cup	160	154	1
chocolate	½ cup	150	140	1
chocolate instant	½ cup	155	130	1
rice	½ cup	155	140	1
tapioca	½ cup	145	140	1
vanilla	½ cup	145	140	1
vanilla instant	½ cup	150	140	1
READY-TO-USE Jell-O				
Chocolate	1 (4 oz)	171	182	1
Chocolate Caramel Swirl	1 (4 oz)	175	169	1
Chocolate Vanilla Light	1 (4 oz)	104	206	1
Chocolate Vanilla Swirl	1 (4 oz)	175	169	1
Chocolate Vanilla Swirl	1 (5.5 oz)	240	249	1
Chocolate Fudge	1 (4 oz)	171	182	1
Chocolate Fudge Light	1 (4 oz)	101	156	1

FOOD	PORTION	CAL	VIT A	VIT C
Jell-O *(cont.)*				
Chocolate Fudge Milk Chocolate Swirl	1 (4 oz)	171	169	1
Chocolate Light	1 (4 oz)	104	192	1
Milk Chocolate	1 (4 oz)	173	181	1
Tapioca	1 (5.5 oz)	229	253	1
Tapioca	1 (4 oz)	167	184	1
Vanilla	1 (4 oz)	182	179	1
Vanilla	1 (5.5 oz)	250	247	1
Vanilla Chocolate Swirl	1 (4 oz)	178	168	1
Vanilla Light	1 (4 oz)	104	220	1
TAKE-OUT				
blancmange	1 serv (4.7 oz)	154	350	tr
bread pudding	1 serv (6.7 oz)	564	1045	tr
queen of puddings	1 serv (4.4 oz)	266	625	1
rice pudding	1 serv (3 oz)	110	255	1
rice pudding w/ raisins	½ cup	246	161	1
tapioca	½ cup	169	196	1
PUMMELO				
fresh	1	228	0	372
sections	1 cup	71	0	116
PUMPKIN				
CANNED				
pumpkin	½ cup	41	26908	5
FRESH				
cooked, mashed	½ cup	24	1320	6
flowers, cooked	½ cup	10	1162	3
flowers, raw	1	0	39	1
leaves, cooked	½ cup	7	866	tr
leaves, raw	½ cup	4	388	2

FOOD	PORTION	CAL	VIT A	VIT C
raw, cubed	½ cup	15	928	5

PURSLANE

cooked	1 cup	21	2130	12
raw	1 cup	7	568	9

QUAIL
(The vitamin A in quail comes from animal sources.)

FRESH

breast w/o skin, raw	1 (2 oz)	69	21	3
w/ skin, raw	1 quail (3.8 oz)	210	265	7

QUICHE
(The vitamin A in quiche comes from animal ingredients like eggs and cheese, and plant sources like vegetables.)

HOME RECIPE

lorraine	⅙ pie (8-in)	600	1640	tr

TAKE-OUT

cheese	1 slice (3 oz)	283	910	tr
lorraine	1 slice (3 oz)	352	790	tr
mushroom	1 slice (3 oz)	256	745	tr

QUINCE

fresh	1	53	37	14

RADICCHIO

raw, shredded	½ cup	5	5	2

RADISHES

DRIED

chinese	½ cup	157	0	0
daikon	½ cup	157	0	0

FRESH

chinese, raw	1 (12 oz)	62	0	74

FOOD	PORTION	CAL	VIT A	VIT C
chinese, raw, sliced	½ cup	8	0	10
chinese, sliced, cooked	½ cup	13	0	11
daikon, raw	1 (12 oz)	62	0	74
daikon, raw, sliced	½ cup	8	0	10
daikon, sliced, cooked	½ cup	13	0	11
red, raw	10	7	3	10
red, sliced	½ cup	10	4	13
white icicle, raw	1 (½ oz)	2	0	5
white icicle, raw, sliced	½ cup	7	0	15
SPROUTS				
raw	½ cup	8	74	6

RAISINS

FOOD	PORTION	CAL	VIT A	VIT C
Dole Golden	½ cup	260	36	3
Dole Seedless	½ cup	260	7	25
golden seedless	1 cup	437	64	5
seedless	1 cup	434	11	5
sultanas	1 oz	88	20	0

RASPBERRIES

FOOD	PORTION	CAL	VIT A	VIT C
CANNED				
in heavy syrup	½ cup	117	43	11
FRESH				
raspberries	1 cup	61	160	31
raspberries	1 pint	154	406	78
FROZEN				
Red (Big Valley)	3.5 oz	55	200	30
Whole in Lite Syrup (Birds Eye)	½ cup	100	100	24
sweetened	1 cup	256	149	41
sweetened	1 pkg (10 oz)	291	169	47

FOOD	PORTION	CAL	VIT A	VIT C
JUICE				
Dole Pure & Light	6 oz	90	33	2
Smucker's	8 oz	120	100	12
RED BEANS				
CANNED				
Green Giant	½ cup	90	0	0
Hunt's Small	4 oz	90	tr	1
Van Camp's	1 cup	194	0	0
RELISH				
cranberry orange	½ cup	246	97	25
hamburger	1 tbsp	19	40	tr
hamburger	½ cup	158	325	3
hot dog	1 tbsp	14	25	tr
hot dog	½ cup	111	203	1
sweet	1 tbsp	19	23	tr
sweet	½ cup	159	189	1
RHUBARB				
Big Valley, frzn	3.5 oz	16	100	9
fresh	½ cup	13	61	5
frzn	½ cup	60	73	3
frzn, as prep w/ sugar	½ cup	139	83	4

RICE
(The vitamin A in prepared rice dishes comes from animal
ingredients like cheese and meat, and from plant sources
like tomato sauce and vegetables.)

FOOD	PORTION	CAL	VIT A	VIT C
CANNED				
Van Camp's Spanish	1 cup	160	1228	1
DRY MIX				
Knorr Risotto Tomato	½ cup	110	300	15

FOOD	PORTION	CAL	VIT A	VIT C
Knorr Risotto With Peas And Corn	½ cup	110	100	6
Lipton Golden Saute				
Fried Rice Beef	½ cup	124	191	tr
Fried Rice Chicken	½ cup	129	5	tr
Fried Rice Oriental	½ cup	127	32	tr
Lipton Rice And Sauce				
Beef	½ cup	119	208	1
Cajun	½ cup	123	195	3
Cheddar Broccoli	½ cup	125	68	2
Chicken	½ cup	124	176	1
Chicken Broccoli	½ cup	129	509	4
Creamy Chicken	½ cup	142	1102	1
Herbs & Butter	½ cup	123	48	0
Long Grain Wild Rice Original	½ cup	121	0	tr
Mushroom	½ cup	123	0	1
Pilaf	½ cup	122	0	0
Skillet Style, Spanish	½ cup	104	234	6
Spanish	½ cup	118	256	3
Lipton Rice Asparagus With Hollandaise	½ cup	123	66	1
Minute Long Grain And Wild, as prep	½ cup	149	154	1
Minute Microwave Broccoli Almondin	½ cup	143	165	2
Minute Microwave Cheddar Cheese Broccoli	½ cup	164	218	2
Minute Microwave French Pilaf	½ cup	133	117	tr
Minute Microwave Long Grain Brown And Wild	½ cup	140	109	tr
Minute Microwave Rice With Savory Cheese Sauce, as prep	½ cup	162	154	tr

FOOD	PORTION	CAL	VIT A	VIT C
Rice-A-Roni				
Beef & Mushroom	½ cup	150	200	1
Chicken	½ cup	150	200	1
Chicken & Broccoli	½ cup	150	200	1
Chicken & Vegetables	½ cup	140	750	1
Long Grain & Wild Original	½ cup	130	300	5
Spanish	½ cup	150	500	15
Yellow Rice	½ cup	140	100	0
Ultra Slim-Fast Oriental Style	2.3 oz	240	750	18
Ultra Slim-Fast Rice & Chicken Sauce	2.3 oz	240	750	18
FROZEN				
Birds Eye Rice and Broccoli Au Gratin	½ pkg	150	500	6
Budget Gourmet Oriental Rice With Vegetables	1 pkg	240	1000	9
Budget Gourmet Rice Mexicana	1 pkg	240	3000	4
Budget Gourmet Rice Pilaf With Green Beans	1 pkg	240	400	9
Green Giant				
Garden Gourmet Asparagus Pilaf	1 pkg	190	3000	12
Garden Gourmet Sherry Wild Rice	1 pkg	210	300	5
One Serve Rice 'N Broccoli in Cheese Sauce	1 pkg	180	2500	18
One Serve Rice, Peas And Mushrooms With Sauce	1 pkg	130	100	4
Rice Originals Italian Rice & Spinach in Cheese Sauce	½ cup	140	500	0
Rice Originals Pilaf	½ cup	110	0	0
Rice Originals Rice 'N Broccoli in Cheese Sauce	½ cup	120	1000	6

FOOD	PORTION	CAL	VIT A	VIT C
Green Giant *(cont.)*				
Rice Originals Rice Medley	½ cup	100	0	0
Rice Originals White And Wild	½ cup	130	0	0
TAKE-OUT				
pilaf	½ cup	84	726	15
risotto	6.6 oz	426	730	tr
spanish	¾ cup	363	763	26
white				

ROLL

(The vitamin A in rolls comes from animal ingredients like eggs and milk or from plant sources.)

FOOD	PORTION	CAL	VIT A	VIT C
HOME RECIPE				
dinner, as prep w/ 2% milk	1 (2.5 in)	111	118	tr
dinner, as prep w/ whole milk	1 (2.5 in)	112	108	tr
raisin & nut	1 (2 oz)	196	233	tr
MIX				
Hot Roll Mix	2	240	200	0
Pillsbury ready-to-eat cinnamon raisin	1 (2.75 in)	223	129	1
hard	1 (3.5 in)	167	0	0
hot cross bun	1	202	220	0
kaiser	1 (3.5 in)	167	0	0
submarine	1 (4.7 oz)	155	0	0
wheat	1 (1 oz)	77	0	0
whole wheat	(1 (1 oz)	75	0	0
REFRIGERATED				
Pillsbury Best Quick Cinnamon Rolls w/ Icing	1	110	0	0
Pillsbury Butterflake	1	140	0	0
Pillsbury Crescent	1	100	0	0
crescent	1 (1 oz)	98	0	0

FOOD	PORTION	CAL	VIT A	VIT C
ROSE APPLE				
fresh	3.5 oz	32	tr	22
ROSELLE				
fresh	1 cup	28	163	7
ROSEMARY				
dried	1 tsp	4	38	1
RUTABAGA				
FRESH				
cooked, mashed	½ cup	41	0	26
raw, cubed	½ cup	25	0	18
SAGE				
ground	1 tsp	2	41	tr

SALAD
(Some of the vitamin A in salads may be from animal ingredients like meat, cheese or eggs, but most comes from plant sources.)

FOOD	PORTION	CAL	VIT A	VIT C
TAKE-OUT				
chef w/o dressing	1½ cups	386	1197	15
tossed w/o dressing	1½ cups	32	2352	48
tossed w/o dressing	¾ cup	16	1182	24
tossed w/o dressing w/ cheese & egg	1½ cups	102	822	10
tossed w/o dressing w/ chicken	1½ cups	105	935	17
tossed w/o dressing w/ pasta & seafood	1½ cups (14.6 oz)	380	6245	38
tossed w/o dressing w/ shrimp	1½ cups	107	791	9
waldorf	½ cup	79	125	2

FOOD	PORTION	CAL	VIT A	VIT C
SALAD DRESSING				
HOME RECIPE				
french	1 tbsp	88	72	tr
MIX				
Good Seasons Classic Dill	1 pkg	28	27	tr
READY-TO-USE				
Healthy Sensation				
Blue Cheese	1 tbsp	19	6	0
French	1 tbsp	21	9	tr
Honey Dijon	1 tbsp	26	tr	tr
Italian	1 tbsp	7	117	1
Ranch	1 tbsp	15	7	tr
Thousand Island	1 tbsp	20	20	tr
Italian	1 tbsp	7	117	1
Ultra Slim-Fast French	1 tbsp	20	500	6
Ultra Slim-Fast Italian	1 tbsp	6	500	6
Wishbone				
Blue Cheese Chunky	1 tbsp	73	6	0
Blue Cheese Chunky Lite	1 tbsp	40	0	0
Caesar With Olive Oil Lite	1 tbsp	28	3	tr
Dijon Vinaigrette Classic	1 tbsp	57	132	2
Dijon Vinaigrette Classic Lite	1 tbsp	30	0	0
French Deluxe	1 tbsp	57	12	tr
French Lite	1 tbsp	30	0	0
French Red	1 tbsp	64	1646	1
French Red Lite	1 tbsp	17	289	tr
French Sweet 'N Spicy	1 tbsp	613	42	1
French Sweet 'N Spicy Lite	1 tbsp	17	25	tr
Italian	1 tbsp	45	20	1
Italian Creamy	1 tbsp	54	28	1
Italian Creamy Lite	1 tbsp	26	0	0

FOOD	PORTION	CAL	VIT A	VIT C
Italian Lite	1 tbsp	6	8	tr
Italian Robusto	1 tbsp	46	31	1
Olive Oil Italian Classic	1 tbsp	33	10	tr
Olive Oil Italian Classic Lite	1 tbsp	20	0	0
Olive Oil Vinaigrette	1 tbsp	30	1	0
Olive Oil Vinaigrette Lite	1 tbsp	16	2	0
Ranch	1 tbsp	76	9	tr
Ranch Lite	1 tbsp	42	0	0
Red Wine Olive Oil Vinaigrette	1 tbsp	34	10	1
Russian	1 tbsp	54	50	1
Russian Lite	1 tbsp	21	0	0
Thousand Island	1 tbsp	66	37	1
Thousand Island Lite	1 tbsp	22	0	0
blue cheese	1 tbsp	77	32	tr
russian	1 tbsp	76	106	1

SALMON
(The vitamin A in salmon comes from animal sources.)

FOOD	PORTION	CAL	VIT A	VIT C
CANNED				
Deming's Alaska Keta	½ cup	140	0	0
Humpty Dumpty Alaska Chum	½ cup	140	0	0
pink w/ bone	1 can (15.9 oz)	631	250	0
pink w/ bone	3 oz	118	47	0
sockeye w/ bone	1 can (12.9 oz)	566	648	0
sockeye w/ bone	3 oz	130	149	0
TAKE-OUT				
salmon cake	1 (3 oz)	241	446	tr

SALSA

FOOD	PORTION	CAL	VIT A	VIT C
Casa Fiesta Chili Salsa	1 oz	9	67	tr
Rosarita Chunky Hot	3 tbsp (1.5 oz)	25	92	17

FOOD	PORTION	CAL	VIT A	VIT C
Rosarita Chunky Medium	3 tbsp (1.5 oz)	25	94	17
Rosarita Chunky Mild	3 tbsp (1.5 oz)	25	91	17
Rosarita Taco Salsa Chunky Medium	3 tbsp (1.5 oz)	25	87	16
Rosarita Taco Salsa Chunky Mild	3 tbsp (1.5 oz)	25	80	16

SALSIFY

FRESH

cooked slices	½ cup	46	0	3
raw, sliced	½ cup	55	0	5

SALT/SEASONED SALT

salt	1 tsp	0	0	0

SAPODILLA

fresh	1	140	102	25
fresh, cut up	1 cup	199	145	35

SAPOTES

fresh	1	301	923	45

SARDINES
(The vitamin A in sardines comes mainly from animal sources; the exception would be tomato sauce, a rich plant source.)

CANNED

pacific in tomato sauce w/ bone	1	68	139	tr
pacific in tomato sauce w/ bone	1 can (13 oz)	658	1351	4

SAUCE
(The vitamin A in sauces can come either from animal sources like eggs or from plant sources like tomatoes.)

FOOD	PORTION	CAL	VIT A	VIT C
DRY				
Etoufee Seasoning Mix (Cajun King)	3.5 oz	383	4660	20
Hollandaise, as prep (Knorr)	2 oz	170	500	1
Jambalaya Seasoning Mix (Cajun King)	3.5 oz	375	2150	16
Napoli, as prep (Knorr)	4 oz	100	1750	42
JARRED				
Bandito Diavalo Spicy (Newman's Own)	4 oz	70	750	12
Hunt's				
Barbecue Homestyle	1 tbsp	20	15	2
Barbecue Original	1 tbsp	20	16	2
Barbecue Southern Style	1 tbsp	20	15	2
Barbecue Country Style	1 tbsp	20	15	2
Barbecue Hickory	1 tbsp	20	15	2
Barbecue Kansas City Style	1 tbsp	20	15	2
Barbecue New Orleans Style	1 tbsp	20	11	2
Barbecue Texas Style	1 tbsp	25	18	2
Barbecue Western Style	1 tbsp	20	15	2
Barbecue Thick & Rich Chunky (Heinz)	1 oz	30	400	1
Barbecue Thick & Rich Hickory Smoke (Heinz)	1 oz	35	200	1
Barbecue Thick & Rich Mesquite Smoke (Heinz)	1 oz	30	300	1
Barbecue Thick & Rich Texas Hot (Heinz)	1 oz	30	200	1
Cajun Style (Golden Dipt)	1 oz	90	100	4
Cocktail (Sauceworks)	1 tbsp	14	100	1
Enchilada Sauce (Gebhardt)	3 tbsp (1.5 oz)	25	45	1
Hot Dog (Just Rite)	2 oz	60	5	2
Manwich Mexican	2.5 oz	35	200	2

FOOD	PORTION	CAL	VIT A	VIT C
Seafood Cocktail (Golden Dipt)	1 tbsp	20	100	4
Seafood Cocktail Extra Hot (Golden Dipt)	1 tbsp	20	200	4
Sloppy Joe (Manwich)	2.5 oz	40	150	5
Tabasco (McIlhenny)	¼ tsp	tr	7	tr
barbecue	1 cup	188	2170	18
teriyaki	1 oz	30	0	0
teriyaki	1 tbsp	15	0	0

SAUERKRAUT

canned	½ cup	22	21	17

SAUSAGE

TAKE-OUT

pork	1 link (.5 oz)	48	tr	0
pork	1 patty (1 oz)	100	tr	0

SAUSAGE DISHES
(The vitamin A in sausage dishes comes from animal ingredients and plant ingredients.)

sausage roll	1 (2.3 oz)	311	405	0

SCALLOP
(The vitamin A in prepared scallops comes from animal and plant ingredients.)

breaded & fried	6 (5 oz)	386	139	0

SCONE
(The vitamin A in scones comes from animal and plant ingredients.)

cheese	1 (1.75 oz)	182	425	tr
plain	1 (1.75 oz)	181	350	tr

SEAWEED

DRIED

agar	1 oz	87	0	0

FOOD	PORTION	CAL	VIT A	VIT C
FRESH				
agar	1 oz	tr	0	0
laver	1 oz	10	1483	11
nori	1 oz	10	1483	11
wakame	1 oz	13	103	1
SESAME				
seeds, dried	1 cup	825	13	0
seeds, dried	1 tbsp	52	1	0
sesame butter	1 tbsp	95	8	0
SESBANIA				
flower	1	1	0	2
flowers	1 cup	5	0	15
flowers, cooked	1 cup	23	0	39
SHELLIE BEANS				
CANNED				
shellie beans	½ cup	37	278	4
SHERBET				
(The vitamin A in sherbet comes mostly from plant sources, with a lesser amount from animal sources.)				
orange	1 cup	270	185	4
orange	½ gal	2158	1480	31
SHRIMP				
READY-TO-USE				
Fried Shrimp (American Original Foods)	4 oz	253	150	1
TAKE-OUT				
breaded & fried	6 to 8 (6 oz)	454	119	0
jambalaya	¾ cup	188	1256	19
SNACKS				
Health Valley Cheddar Lites	0.75 oz	40	29	tr

FOOD	PORTION	CAL	VIT A	VIT C
Ultra Slim-Fast Lite N' Tasty Cheese Curls	1 oz	110	500	6

SNAP BEANS

CANNED

green	½ cup	13	237	3
green, low sodium	½ cup	13	237	3
italian	½ cup	13	237	3
italian, low sodium	½ cup	13	237	3
yellow	½ cup	13	237	3
yellow, low sodium	½ cup	13	237	3

FRESH

green, cooked	½ cup	22	413	6
green, raw	½ cup	17	368	9
yellow, raw	½ cup	17	50	9
yellow, cooked	½ cup	22	50	6

FROZEN

green, cooked	½ cup	18	359	6
italian, cooked	½ cup	18	359	6
yellow, cooked	½ cup	18	359	6

SODA
(Yoo-Hoo is made with milk, an animal source; Orangina is made with fruit juice, a vegetable source.)

Lucozade	7 oz	136	0	0
Orangina	6 fl oz	80	0	6
Yoo-Hoo	9 fl oz	150	500	6
club	12 oz	0	0	0
cola	12 oz	151	0	0
cream	12 oz	191	0	0
diet cola	12 oz	2	0	0
diet cola w/ Nutrasweet	12 oz	2	0	0

FOOD	PORTION	CAL	VIT A	VIT C
diet cola w/ saccharin	12 oz	2	0	0
ginger ale	12 oz can	124	0	0
grape	12 oz	161	0	0
lemon lime	12 oz	149	0	0
orange	12 oz	177	0	0
pepper type	12 oz	151	0	0
quinine	12 oz	125	0	0
root beer	12 oz	152	0	0
tonic water	12 oz	125	0	0

SOLE
FRESH

raw	3½ oz	90	tr	0

SOUFFLE
(The vitamin A in soufflés can come from animal ingredients like eggs and cheese, or from plant sources like spinach.)

HOME RECIPE

cheese	3.5 oz	253	1215	tr
spinach	1 cup	218	3461	3

SOUP
(The vitamin A in soups can come from animal sources like chicken and beef or from plant sources like vegetables).

CANNED

Asparagus Cream of, as prep (Campbell)	8 oz	80	200	1
Bean And Ham (Healthy Choice)	½ can (7.5 oz)	220	300	2
Bean Homestyle, as prep (Campbell)	8 oz	130	750	2
Beef Broth (Health Valley)	7.5 oz	10	1	0
Beef Broth No Salt Added (Health Valley)	7.5 oz	10	1	0

FOOD	PORTION	CAL	VIT A	VIT C
Beef Chunky Ready-To-Serve (Campbell)	10.75 oz	200	5000	6
Beef with Vegetables And Pasta Home Cookin' (Campbell)	10.75	140	200	4
Beef, as prep (Campbell)	8 oz	80	1000	1
Black Bean (Goya)	7.5 oz	160	<100	2
Black Bean (Health Valley)	7.5 oz	150	5112	2
Black Bean No Salt Added (Health Valley)	7.5 oz	150	5112	2
Borscht (Gold's)	8 oz	100	100	12
Broccoli Cream of, as prep (Campbell)	8 oz	80	100	6
Broccoli Cream of, as prep w/ 2% milk (Campbell)	8 oz	140	300	6
Chicken Minestrone Home Cookin' (Campbell)	10.75 oz	180	2000	2
Chicken Vegetable Beef Low Sodium Ready-To-Serve (Campbell)	10.75 oz	180	5000	9
Chicken Vegetable Chunky Ready-To-Serve (Campbell)	9.5 oz	170	6500	5
Chicken Broth (Health Valley)	7.5 oz	35	tr	tr
Chicken Broth No Salt Added (Health Valley)	7.5 oz	35	tr	tr
Chicken Noodle Homestyle, as prep (Campbell)	8 oz	70	750	1
Chicken Nuggets w/ Vegetables & Noodles Chunky (Campbell)	10.75 oz	190	2500	9
Chicken With Noodles Low Sodium Ready-To-Serve (Campbell)	10.75 oz	170	1750	2
Chicken With Rice Chunky Ready-To-Serve (Campbell)	9.5 oz	140	6000	4

FOOD	PORTION	CAL	VIT A	VIT C
Chicken With Rice (Healthy Choice)	½ can (7.5 oz)	140	400	6
Chili Beef Chunky Ready-To-Serve (Campbell)	11 oz	290	1250	6
Chili Beef, as prep (Campbell)	8 oz	140	500	2
Chunky Beef Vegetable (Healthy Choice)	½ can (7.5 oz)	110	1000	9
Chunky Chicken Noodle And Vegetable (Healthy Choice)	½ can (7.5 oz)	160	1750	15
Chunky Chicken Vegetable (Health Valley)	7.5 oz	125	3283	1
Chunky Five Bean Vegetable (Health Valley)	7.5 oz	110	5000	3
Chunky Five Bean Vegetable No Salt Added (Health Valley)	7.5 oz	110	5000	3
Chunky Vegetable Chicken No Salt Added (Health Valley)	7.5 oz	125	3283	1
Clam Chowder Manhattan Style Chunky Ready-To-Serve (Campbell)	10.75 oz	160	5500	12
Clam Chowder Manhattan Style, as prep (Campbell)	8 oz	70	1500	5
Clam Chowder New England, as prep w/ whole milk (Campbell)	8 oz	150	100	2
Country Vegetable (Healthy Choice)	½ can (7.5 oz)	120	1000	6
Country Vegetable Home Cookin' (Campbell)	10¾ oz	120	4500	4
Green Split Pea (Health Valley)	7.5 oz	180	5122	1
Green Split Pea No Salt Added (Health Valley)	7.5 oz	180	5122	1
Ham 'n Butter Bean Chunky Ready-To-Serve (Campbell)	10¾ oz	280	3000	6
Hearty Beef (Healthy Choice)	½ can (7.5 oz)	120	750	9

FOOD	PORTION	CAL	VIT A	VIT C
Hearty Chicken (Healthy Choice)	½ can (7.5 oz)	150	1000	2
Hearty Chicken Vegetable Healthy Request (Campbell)	8 oz	120	500	1
Hearty Lentil Home Cookin' (Campbell)	10¾ oz	170	4000	4
Lentil (Health Valley)	7.5 oz	220	5132	1
Lentil No Salt Added (Health Valley)	7.5 oz	220	5132	1
Manhattan Clam Chowder (Health Valley)	7.5 oz	110	5106	3
Manhattan Clam Chowder No Salt Added (Health Valley)	7.5 oz	110	5106	3
Manhattan Clam Chowder, as prep w/ water (Snow's)	7.5 fl oz	70	2000	1
Mediterranean Vegetable Chunky Ready-To-Serve (Campbell)	9.5 oz	170	5500	6
Minestrone (Health Valley)	7.5 oz	130	5010	1
Minestrone (Healthy Choice)	½ can (7.5 oz)	160	300	15
Minestrone Chunky Ready-To-Serve (Campbell)	9.5 oz	160	4500	6
Minestrone Home Cookin' (Campbell)	10.75 oz	140	4500	5
Minestrone No Salt Added (Health Valley)	7.5 oz	130	5010	1
Minestrone, as prep (Campbell)	8 oz	80	2250	4
Mushroom Barley (Health Valley)	7.5 oz	100	5325	3
Mushroom Barley No Salt Added (Health Valley)	7.5 oz	100	5325	3
Nacho Cheese, as prep (Campbell)	8 oz	110	1250	6
Nacho Cheese, as prep w/ milk (Campbell)	8 oz	180	1500	6

FOOD	PORTION	CAL	VIT A	VIT C
New England Chowder (American Original Foods)	4 oz	64	tr	2
New England Chowder, as prep w/ milk (American Original Foods)	4 oz	145	150	4
Old Fashioned Bean w/ Ham Chunky Ready-To-Serve (Campbell)	11 oz	290	4500	6
Old Fashioned Chicken Chunky Ready-To-Serve (Campbell)	10.75 oz	180	6000	6
Old Fashioned Chicken Noodle (Healthy Choice)	½ can (7.5 oz)	90	400	12
Old Fashioned Vegetable Beef Chunky Ready-To-Serve (Campbell)	10.75 oz	190	5500	6
Oyster Stew, as prep w/ whole milk (Campbell)	8 oz	140	100	6
Pepper Steak Chunky Ready-To-Serve (Campbell)	10.75 oz	180	2500	9
Potato Leek (Health Valley)	7.5 oz	130	4985	tr
Potato Leek No Salt Added (Health Valley)	7.5 oz	130	4985	tr
Schav (Gold's)	8 oz	25	1250	9
Shrimp Cream Of, as prep w/ whole milk (Campbell)	8 oz	160	200	1
Sirloin Burger Chunky Ready-To-Serve (Campbell)	10.75 oz	220	4500	6
Split Pea And Ham (Healthy Choice)	½ can (7.5 oz)	170	500	6
Split Pea Low Sodium Ready-To-Serve (Campbell)	10.75 oz	230	1500	5
Split Pea with Ham Home Cookin' (Campbell)	10.75 oz	230	2500	6
Split Pea w/ Ham Chunky Ready-To-Serve (Campbell)	10.75 oz	230	3500	6
Tomato (Health Valley)	7.5 oz	130	4952	21

FOOD	PORTION	CAL	VIT A	VIT C
Tomato Bisque, as prep (Campbell)	8 oz	120	500	18
Tomato Garden (Healthy Choice)	½ can (7.5 oz)	130	500	6
Tomato Garden Home Cookin' (Campbell)	10.75 oz	150	2750	12
Tomato Healthy Request, as prep (Campbell)	8 oz	90	400	27
Tomato Healthy Request, as prep w/ skim milk (Campbell)	8 oz	130	750	27
Tomato Homestyle Cream Of, as prep (Campbell)	8 oz	110	500	24
Tomato Homestyle Cream Of, as prep w/ whole milk (Campbell)	8 oz	180	750	24
Tomato No Salt Added (Health Valley)	7.5 oz	130	4952	21
Tomato Rice Old Fashioned, as prep (Campbell)	8 oz	110	40	12
Tomato with Tomato Pieces Low Sodium Ready-To-Serve (Campbell)	10.75 oz	190	1500	35
Tomato Zesty, as prep (Campbell)	8 oz	100	1250	18
Tomato, as prep (Campbell)	8 oz	90	500	27
Tomato, as prep w/ 2% milk (Campbell)	8 oz	150	750	27
Turkey Vegetable Chunky Ready-To-Serve (Campbell)	9¾ oz	150	6500	6
Vegetable (Health Valley)	7.5 oz	110	5000	3
Vegetable Healthy Request, as prep (Campbell)	8 oz	90	2000	2
Vegetable Homestyle, as prep (Campbell)	8 oz	60	2250	4
Vegetable Beef (Healthy Choice)	½ can (7.5 oz)	130	500	15

FOOD	PORTION	CAL	VIT A	VIT C
Vegetable Beef Home Cookin' (Campbell)	10.75 oz	140	5000	9
Vegetable Beef, as prep (Campbell)	8 oz	70	2000	2
Vegetable Chunky Ready-To-Serve (Campbell)	10.75 oz	160	6500	5
Vegetable No Salt Added (Health Valley)	7.5 oz	110	5000	3
Vegetable Old Fashioned, as prep (Campbell)	8 oz	60	2500	1
Vegetable, as prep (Campbell)	8 oz	90	2000	4
Vegetarian Vegetable, as prep (Campbell)	8 oz	80	2000	4
asparagus, cream of, as prep w/ milk	1 cup	161	599	4
asparagus, cream of, as prep w/ water	1 cup	87	445	3
beef broth, ready-to-serve	1 can (14 oz)	27	0	0
beef broth, ready-to-serve	1 cup	16	0	0
beef noodle, as prep w/ water	1 cup	84	629	tr
black bean turtle soup	1 cup	218	10	6
black bean, as prep w/ water	1 cup	116	506	1
celery, cream of, as prep w/ water	1 cup	90	306	tr
celery, cream of, as prep w/ milk	1 cup	165	461	1
celery cream of, not prep	1 can (10.75 oz)	219	746	1
cheese, not prep	1 can (11 oz)	377	2643	0
cheese, as prep w/ milk	1 cup	230	1243	1
cheese, as prep w/ water	1 cup	155	1088	0
chicken broth, as prep w/ water	1 cup	39	0	0
chicken, cream of, as prep w/ milk	1 cup	191	715	1

FOOD	PORTION	CAL	VIT A	VIT C
chicken, cream of, as prep w/ water	1 cup	116	560	tr
chicken gumbo, as prep w/ water	1 cup	56	136	5
chicken noodle, as prep w/ water	1 cup	75	711	tr
chicken rice, as prep w/ water	1 cup	251	660	tr
clam chowder, Manhattan, as prep w/ water	1 cup	77	963	4
clam chowder, New England, as prep w/ milk	1 cup	163	164	4
clam chowder, New England, as prep w/ water	1 cup	95	8	2
consomme w/ gelatin, as prep w/ water	1 cup	29	0	1
consomme w/ gelatin, not prep	1 can (10½ oz)	71	0	2
french onion, as prep w/ water	1 cup	57	0	1
gazpacho, ready-to-serve	1 cup	57	200	3
minestrone, as prep w/ water	1 cup	83	2337	1
mushroom, cream of, as prep w/ milk	1 cup	203	154	2
mushroom, cream of, as prep w/ water	1 cup	129	0	1
oyster stew, as prep w/ milk	1 cup	134	225	4
oyster stew, as prep w/ water	1 cup	59	71	3
pepperpot, as prep w/ water	1 cup	103	856	1
potato, cream of, as prep w/ water	1 cup	73	288	0
potato, cream of, as prep w/ milk	1 cup	148	443	1
scotch broth, as prep w/ water	1 cup	80	2180	1
split pea w/ ham, as prep w/ water	1 cup	189	444	1

FOOD	PORTION	CAL	VIT A	VIT C
tomato, as prep w/ milk	1 cup	160	849	68
tomato, as prep w/ water	1 cup	86	688	67
vegetarian vegetable, as prep w/ water	1 cup	72	3005	1
vichyssoise	1 cup	148	443	1
DRY				
Asparagus, as prep (Knorr)	8 oz	80	100	5
Bean With Bacon 'n Ham Microwave (Campbell)	7.5 oz	230	750	1
Beef Instant Oriental Noodle (Lipton)	8 oz	177	895	4
Beef Mushroom (Lipton)	8 oz	38	0	1
Beef Noodle (Campbell's Cup)	1 (1.35 oz)	130	1250	1
Beef Noodle (Ultra Slim-Fast)	6 oz	45	500	6
Beef With Vegetables Low Fat, as prep (Cup-A-Ramen)	8 oz	220	2000	1
Beefy Onion (Lipton)	8 oz	27	0	1
Chick 'N Pasta, as prep (Knorr)	8 oz	90	1250	6
Chicken Vegetable (Cup-A-Soup)	6 oz	47	366	8
Chicken Broth (Cup-A-Soup)	6 oz	19	0	0
Chicken Instant Oriental Noodle (Lipton)	8 oz	180	1165	31
Chicken Leek (Ultra Slim-Fast)	6 oz	50	500	6
Chicken Noodle (Lipton)	8 oz	82	19	tr
Chicken Noodle (Ultra Slim-Fast)	6 oz	45	500	6
Chicken Noodle Hearty (Lipton)	8 oz	81	37	0
Chicken with Vegetables Low Fat, as prep (Cup-A-Ramen)	8 oz	220	2000	1
Chicken with Vegetables, as prep (Cup-A-Ramen)	8 oz	270	1000	1

FOOD	PORTION	CAL	VIT A	VIT C
Chili Beef Microwave (Campbell)	7.5 oz	190	1000	1
Country Vegetable (Lipton)	8 oz	80	2778	2
Country Barley, as prep (Knorr)	8 oz	120	1250	9
Creamy Broccoli (Ultra Slim-Fast)	6 oz	75	500	6
Creamy Broccoli And Cheese (Cup-A-Soup)	6 oz	70	103	1
Creamy Tomato (Ultra Slim-Fast)	6 oz	60	500	6
Fine Herb, as prep (Knorr)	8 oz	130	990	12
Giggle Noodle (Lipton)	8 oz	72	5	tr
Green Pea (Cup-A-Soup)	6 oz	113	94	tr
Hearty Minestrone, as prep (Knorr)	10 oz	130	750	24
Hearty Chicken And Noodles (Cup-A-Soup)	6 oz	110	702	0
Hearty Creamy Chicken Lots-A-Noodles (Cup-A-Soup)	7 oz	179	0	0
Hearty Noodles With Vegetables (Campbell's Cup)	1 (1.7 oz)	180	750	1
Hearty Noodles With Vegetables (Lipton)	8 oz	75	442	0
Hearty Vegetable (Ultra Slim-Fast)	6 oz	50	500	6
Mushroom, Cream of (Cup-A-Soup)	6 oz	71	0	tr
Onion (Cup-A-Soup)	6 oz	27	0	1
Onion (Lipton)	8 oz	20	0	tr
Onion (Ultra Slim-Fast)	6 oz	45	500	6
Onion Golden (Lipton)	8 oz	62	0	0
Onion Mushroom (Lipton)	8 oz	41	0	1

FOOD	PORTION	CAL	VIT A	VIT C
Oriental With Vegetables Low Fat, as prep (Cup-A-Ramen)	8 oz	220	2000	1
Oriental With Vegetables, as prep (Cup-A-Ramen)	8 oz	270	750	1
Oxtail Hearty Beef, as prep (Knorr)	8 oz	70	200	12
Potato Leek (Ultra Slim-Fast)	6 oz	80	500	6
Ring-O-Noodle (Lipton)	8 oz	67	5	tr
Shrimp With Vegetables Low Fat, as prep (Cup-A-Ramen)	8 oz	230	1250	1
Shrimp With Vegetables, as prep (Cup-A-Ramen)	8 oz	280	1500	2
Tomato (Cup-A-Soup)	6 oz	103	467	5
Tomato Basil, as prep (Knorr)	8 oz	90	1250	54
Vegetable (Lipton)	8 oz	37	2231	2
Vegetable Beef Microwave (Campbell)	7½ oz	100	1250	2
Vegetable, as prep (Knorr)	8 oz	35	1250	12
chicken broth	1 pkg (0./2 oz)	16	30	tr
chicken broth, as prep w/ water	1 cup	21	40	tr
chicken noodle, as prep w/ water	1 cup	53	63	tr
french onion, not prep	1 pkg (1.4 oz)	115	8	1
onion, as prep w/ water	1 cup	28	2	tr
tomato, as prep w/ water	1 cup	102	832	5
FROZEN Kettle Ready				
Asparagus, Cream Of	6 oz	62	284	2
Black Bean With Ham	6 oz	154	698	9
Boston Clam Chowder	6 oz	131	301	3
Broccoli, Cream Of	6 oz	94	584	15
Cauliflower, Cream Of	6 oz	93	630	8

FOOD	PORTION	CAL	VIT A	VIT C
Kettle Ready *(cont.)*				
Cheddar Broccoli, Cream Of	6 oz	137	708	15
Chicken, Cream Of	6 oz	98	317	1
Chicken Gumbo	6 oz	94	187	10
Chicken Noodle	6 oz	94	821	1
Chili	6 oz	161	468	3
Corn & Broccoli Chowder	6 oz	102	323	12
Creamy Cheddar	6 oz	158	251	0
French Onion	6 oz	42	82	2
Garden Vegetable	6 oz	85	1646	9
Hearty Minestrone	6 oz	104	1794	11
Hearty Beef Vegetable	6 oz	85	1212	8
Manhattan Clam Chowder	6 oz	69	1222	15
Mushroom, Cream Of	6 oz	85	264	0
New England Clam Chowder	6 oz	116	570	3
Potato, Cream Of	6 oz	121	580	9
Savory Bean With Ham	6 oz	113	222	11
Split Pea With Ham	6 oz	155	470	11
Tomato Florentine	6 oz	106	889	4
Tortellini In Tomato	6 oz	122	237	2
HOME RECIPE				
black bean turtle soup	1 cup	241	11	0
corn & cheese chowder	¾ cup	215	636	7
greek	¾ cup	63	39	4
SHELF STABLE				
Chunky Beef Vegetable (Healthy Choice)	7.5 oz cup	110	1000	9
Chunky Chicken Noodle & Vegetable (Healthy Choice)	7.5 oz cup	160	1750	15
TAKE-OUT				
oxtail	5 oz	64	0	0

FOOD	PORTION	CAL	VIT A	VIT C

SOUR CREAM
(The vitamin A in sour cream comes from animal sources.)

FOOD	PORTION	CAL	VIT A	VIT C
sour cream	1 cup	493	1817	2
sour cream	1 tbsp	26	95	tr

SOUR CREAM SUBSTITUTES

nondairy	1 cup	479	0	0
nondairy	1 oz	59	0	0

SOURSOP

fresh	1	416	18	129
fresh, cut up	1 cup	150	5	46

SOY

soy milk	1 cup	79	77	0
soy sauce	1 tbsp	7	0	0
soy sauce shoyu	1 tbsp	9	0	0
soy sauce tamari	1 tbsp	11	0	0
soya cheese	1.4 oz	128	0	0
soybean sprouts, raw	½ cup	43	4	5
soybean sprouts, steamed	½ cup	38	5	4
soybean sprouts, stir fried	1 cup	125	17	12
soybeans, cooked	1 cup	298	15	3
soybeans, dry-roasted	½ cup	387	20	4
soybeans, roasted	½ cup	405	172	2
soybeans, roasted & toasted	1 cup	490	216	2
soybeans, roasted & toasted	1 oz	129	57	1
soybeans, salted, roasted & toasted	1 cup	490	216	2
soybeans, salted, roasted & toasted	1 oz	129	57	1

FOOD	PORTION	CAL	VIT A	VIT C
SPAGHETTI SAUCE				
JARRED				
Hunt's				
Chunky	4 oz	50	60	9
Homestyle	4 oz	60	100	12
Homestyle With Meat	4 oz	60	146	18
Homestyle With Mushrooms	4 oz	50	150	18
Traditional	4 oz	70	100	9
With Meat	4 oz	70	156	18
With Mushrooms	4 oz	70	100	9
Newman's Own	4 oz	70	750	12
Newman's Own Sockarooni	4 oz	70	750	12
Newman's Own With Mushrooms	4 oz	70	750	12
Prego				
Chunky Sausage & Green Peppers	4 oz	160	1000	18
Extra Chunky Garden Combination	4 oz	80	1000	24
Extra Chunky Mushroom And Green Pepper	4 oz	100	750	12
Extra Chunky Mushroom And Onion	4 oz	100	500	12
Extra Chunky Mushroom And Tomato	4 oz	110	500	12
Extra Chunky Mushroom With Extra Spice	4 oz	100	750	21
Extra Chunky Tomato And Onion	4 oz	110	500	12
Marinara	4 oz	100	750	18
Meat Flavored	4 oz	140	1000	15
Mushroom	4 oz	130	1000	15

FOOD	PORTION	CAL	VIT A	VIT C
Onion And Garlic	4 oz	110	1000	5
Regular	4 oz	130	1000	18
Three Cheese	4 oz	100	750	21
Tomato & Basil	4 oz	100	1000	21
Ragu				
Chunky Gardenstyle Extra Tomatoes, Garlic & Onions	4 oz	70	750	9
Chunky Gardenstyle Green & Red Peppers	4 oz	70	750	9
Chunky Gardenstyle Italian Garden Combination	4 oz	70	750	9
Chunky Gardenstyle Mushrooms & Onions	4 oz	70	750	9
Homestyle w/ Mushrooms	4 oz	110	300	6
Homestyle w/ Tomato & Herbs	4 oz	110	300	6
Homestyle w/ Meat	4 oz	110	300	6
Italian Cooking Sauce	4 oz	70	500	2
Joe	3.5 oz	50	500	6
Old World Style Marinara	4 oz	80	750	6
Old World Style Pizza	1.6 oz	25	300	5
Old World Style Plain	4 oz	80	750	6
Old World Style w/ Mushrooms	4 oz	80	750	6
Old World Style w/ Meat	4 oz	80	750	6
Thick & Hearty Plain	4 oz	100	750	9
Thick & Hearty w/ Meat	4 oz	120	750	9
Thick & Hearty w/ Mushrooms	4 oz	100	750	9
marinara sauce	1 cup	171	2403	32
spaghetti sauce	1 cup	272	3055	28

FOOD	PORTION	CAL	VIT A	VIT C
TAKE-OUT				
bolognese	5 oz	195	2260	7

SPANISH FOOD
(The vitamin A in Spanish foods comes from animal sources like meat and cheese or from plant sources like tomatoes.)

FOOD	PORTION	CAL	VIT A	VIT C
CANNED				
Enchilada Sauce Mild (Rosarita)	2.5 oz	25	150	6
Enchiladas (Gebhardt)	2	310	25	3
Picante Chunky Hot (Rosarita)	3 tbsp (2 fl oz)	18	45	45
Picante Chunky Medium (Rosarita)	3 tbsp (2 fl oz)	16	45	10
Picante Chunky Mild (Rosarita)	3 tbsp (2 oz)	25	56	33
Picante Mild (Casa Fiesta)	1 oz	9	67	tr
Taco Sauce Mild (Casa Fiesta)	1 oz	9	67	tr
Taco Sauce Thick And Smooth Hot (Ortega)	1 tbsp	8	200	2
Taco Sauce Thick And Smooth Mild (Ortega)	1 tbsp	8	100	2
Tamales (Derby)	2	160	65	1
Tamales (Gebhardt)	2	290	100	2
Tamales Jumbo (Gebhardt)	2	400	139	3
FROZEN				
Banquet Beef Enchilada & Tamale w/ Chili Gravy	10 oz	300	1500	4
Budget Gourmet Beef Mexicana	1 pkg	520	5000	9
Budget Gourmet Chicken Enchilada Suiza	1 pkg	290	100	6
Budget Gourmet Chicken Mexicana	1 pkg	560	5000	12
Budget Gourmet Sirloin Enchilada Ranchero	1 pkg	280	5000	6

FOOD	PORTION	CAL	VIT A	VIT C
Healthy Choice Enchilada Chicken	12.75 oz	330	500	21
Healthy Choice Enchilada Beef	12.75 oz	350	1250	24
Healthy Choice Enchiladas Chicken	9.5 oz	280	400	21
Healthy Choice Fajitas Beef	7 oz	210	500	6
Healthy Choice Fajitas Chicken	7 oz	200	750	9
Le Menu Entree LightStyle Enchiladas Chicken	8 oz	280	100	9
Lean Cuisine Enchanadas Beef and Bean	9.25 oz	240	400	6
Lean Cuisine Enchanadas Chicken	9.9 oz	290	1250	6
Patio Mexican Dinner	13.25 oz	540	150	4
Swanson Enchiladas Beef	13.75 oz	480	1250	4
Swanson Mexican Style Hungry Man	20.25 oz	820	2000	6
MIX				
Masa Harina De Maiz (Quaker)	2 tortillas	137	0	0
Masa Trigo (Quaker)	2 tortillas	149	0	0
Taco Meat Seasoning Mix Mild (Ortega)	1 filled taco	90	750	1
READY-TO-USE				
Taco Shells (Casa Fiesta)	3.5 oz	480	106	tr
tortilla flour w/o salt	1 8-in diam (1.2 oz)	114	0	0
TAKE-OUT				
burrito w/ apple	1 lg (5.4 oz)	484	849	2
burrito w/ apple	1 sm (2.6 oz)	231	405	tr
burrito w/ beans	2 (7.6 oz)	448	332	2
burrito w/ beans & cheese	2 (6.5 oz)	377	1250	2
burrito w/ beans & chili peppers	2 (7.2 oz)	413	205	1
burrito w/ beans & meat	2 (8.1 oz)	508	636	2

FOOD	PORTION	CAL	VIT A	VIT C
burrito w/ beans, cheese & beef	2 (7.1 oz)	331	799	5
burrito w/ beans, cheese & chili peppers	2 (11.8 oz)	663	1596	7
burrito w/ beef	2 (7.7 oz)	523	277	1
burrito w/ beef & chili peppers	2 (7.1 oz)	426	463	2
burrito w/ beef, cheese & chili peppers	2 (10.7 oz)	634	972	4
burrito w/ cherry	1 lg (5.4 oz)	484	849	2
burrito w/ cherry	1 sm (2.6 oz)	231	405	tr
chimichanga w/ beef	1 (6.1 oz)	425	147	5
chimichanga w/ beef & cheese	1 (6.4 oz)	443	540	3
chimichanga w/ beef & red chili peppers	1 (6.7 oz)	424	262	tr
chimichanga w/ beef, cheese & red chili peppers	1 (6.3 oz)	364	702	2
enchilada w/ cheese	1 (5.7 oz)	320	1160	tr
enchilada w/ cheese & beef	1 (6.7 oz)	324	1135	1
enchirito w/ cheese, beef & beans	1 (6.8 oz)	344	1015	5
frijoles w/ cheese	1 cup (5.9 oz)	226	457	2
nachos w/ cheese	6–8 (4 oz)	345	559	1
nachos w/ cheese & jalapeno peppers	6–8 (7.2 oz)	607	461	tr
nachos w/ cheese, beans, ground beef & peppers	6–8 (8.9 oz)	568	3401	5
nachos w/ cinnamon & sugar	6–8 (3.8 oz)	592	108	8
taco	1 sm (6 oz)	370	855	2
taco salad	1½ cups	279	589	4
taco salad w/ chili con carne	1½ cups	288	1573	3
tostada w/ beans & cheese	1 (5.1 oz)	223	622	1
tostada w/ beans, beef & cheese	1 (7.9 oz)	334	1275	4

FOOD	PORTION	CAL	VIT A	VIT C
tostada w/ beef & cheese	1 (5.7 oz)	315	713	3
tostada w/ guacamole	2 (9.2 oz)	360	1752	4

SPINACH

CANNED
S&W Northwest Premium	½ cup	25	5000	12
spinach	½ cup	25	9390	15

FRESH
Dole	3 oz	9	4751	21
cooked	½ cup	21	7371	9
mustard, chopped, cooked	½ cup	14	7380	59
mustard, raw, chopped	½ cup	17	7425	98
new zealand, chopped, cooked	½ cup	11	3260	14
new zealand, raw	½ cup	4	1232	8
raw, chopped	1 pkg (10 oz)	46	13699	57
raw, chopped	½ cup	6	1880	8

FROZEN
Birds Eye Chopped	½ cup	20	7500	27
Birds Eye Creamed	½ cup	90	1500	15
Birds Eye Leaf	½ cup	20	7500	27
Budget Gourmet Au Gratin	1 pkg	160	750	21
Green Giant	½ cup	25	5000	18
Green Giant Creamed	½ cup	70	1750	2
Green Giant Cut Leaf In Butter Sauce	½ cup	40	7000	24
Green Giant Harvest Fresh	½ cup	25	2500	6
cooked	½ cup	27	7395	12

SQUASH

CANNED
crookneck, sliced	½ cup	14	130	3

FOOD	PORTION	CAL	VIT A	VIT C
FRESH				
acorn, cooked & mashed	½ cup	41	315	8
acorn, cubed & baked	½ cup	57	437	11
butternut, baked	½ cup	41	7141	15
crookneck, raw, sliced	½ cup	12	220	5
crookneck, sliced, cooked	½ cup	18	259	5
hubbard, baked	½ cup	51	6156	10
hubbard, cooked, mashed	½ cup	35	4726	8
scallop, raw, sliced	½ cup	12	72	12
scallop, sliced, cooked	½ cup	14	77	10
spaghetti, cooked	½ cup	23	86	3
FROZEN				
Winter Cooked (Birds Eye)	½ cup	45	4500	12
butternut, cooked, mashed	½ cup	47	4007	4
crookneck, sliced, cooked	½ cup	24	187	7

STRAWBERRIES

FOOD	PORTION	CAL	VIT A	VIT C
CANNED				
in heavy syrup	½ cup	117	33	40
FRESH				
strawberries	1 cup	45	41	85
strawberries	1 pint	97	87	182
FROZEN				
sweetened, sliced	1 cup	245	61	106
sweetened, sliced	1 pkg (10 oz)	273	68	118
unsweetened	1 cup	52	66	61
whole, sweetened	1 cup	200	70	101
whole, sweetened	1 pkg (10 oz)	223	78	112
JUICE				
Kool-Aid Koolers	1 (8.45 oz)	136	1	6

FOOD	PORTION	CAL	VIT A	VIT C

STUFFING/DRESSING
(The vitamin A in stuffing can come from animal
ingredients like eggs or from plant sources like vegetables.)

HOME RECIPE

FOOD	PORTION	CAL	VIT A	VIT C
bread, as prep w/ water & fat	½ cup	251	455	tr
bread, as prep w/ water egg & fat	½ cup	107	431	3
plain, as prep	½ cup (3.5 oz)	195	349	2
sausage	½ cup	292	78	2

MIX

FOOD	PORTION	CAL	VIT A	VIT C
Pepperidge Farm Distinctive Classic Chicken	1 oz	110	300	5
Stove Top				
Beef, as prep	½ cup	178	746	1
Chicken With Rice, as prep	½ cup	182	387	1
Chicken, as prep	½ cup	176	386	1
Cornbread, as prep	½ cup	175	432	1
Flex Serve Cornbread, as prep	½ cup	181	350	1
Flex Serve Homestyle Herb, as prep	½ cup	173	345	1
cornbread, as prep	½ cup	179	353	1

SUGAR

FOOD	PORTION	CAL	VIT A	VIT C
brown	1 cup	820	0	0
white	1 cup	770	0	0
white	1 packet (6 g)	25	0	0
white	1 tbsp	45	0	0

SUGAR SUBSTITUTES

FOOD	PORTION	CAL	VIT A	VIT C
S&W Liquid Table Sweetener	⅛ tsp	0	0	0
Sprinkle Sweet	1 tsp	2	0	0
Sweet*10	⅛ tsp	0	0	0

FOOD	PORTION	CAL	VIT A	VIT C

SUGAR-APPLE

fresh	1	146	9	66
fresh, cut up	1 cup	236	15	91

SURF
(The vitamin A in surf comes from animal sources.)

CANNED Surf (American Original Foods)	4 oz	100	100	1
FRESH Surf (American Original Foods)	4 oz	90	100	1

SWAMP CABBAGE

chopped, cooked	½ cup	10	2548	8
raw, chopped	1 cup	11	3528	31

SWEET POTATO

CANNED in syrup	½ cup	106	7014	11
pieces	1 cup	183	15965	53
FRESH baked w/ skin	1 (3.5 oz)	118	24877	28
leaves, cooked	½ cup	11	293	1
mashed	½ cup	172	27968	28
FROZEN Candied Sweet Potatoes (Mrs. Paul's)	4 oz	170	1750	12
Candied Sweets 'N Apples (Mrs. Paul's)	4 oz	160	1250	30
cooked	½ cup	88	14441	8
HOME RECIPE candied	3.5 oz	144	4399	7

FOOD	PORTION	CAL	VIT A	VIT C
SWEETBREADS				
beef, braised	3 oz	230	0	17
SWISS CHARD				
FRESH				
cooked	½ cup	18	2762	16
raw, chopped	½ cup	3	594	5
SWORDFISH				
(The vitamin A in swordfish comes from animal sources.)				
cooked	3 oz	132	117	1
raw	3 oz	103	101	1
SYRUP				
corn	2 tbsp	122	0	0
TAMARIND				
fresh	1	5	1	tr
fresh, cut up	1 cup	287	36	4
TANGERINE				
CANNED				
in juice pack	½ cup	46	1056	43
in light syrup	½ cup	76	1058	25
FRESH				
sections	1 cup	86	1794	60
tangerine	1	37	773	26
JUICE				
Dole Pure & Light	6 oz	100	200	2
canned, sweetened	1 cup	125	1046	55
fresh	1 cup	106	1037	77
frzn, sweetened, as prep	1 cup	110	1382	58
frzn, sweetened, not prep	6 oz	344	4310	182

FOOD	PORTION	CAL	VIT A	VIT C
TARO				
chips	1 oz	141	0	1
leaves, cooked	½ cup	18	3136	26
raw sliced	½ cup	56	0	2
sliced, cooked	½ cup (2.3 oz)	94	0	3
tahitian, sliced, cooked	½ cup	30	1200	26
TEA/HERBAL TEA				
REGULAR				
Lipton Iced Tea Lemon w/ Vitamin C	6 oz	58	0	22
Lipton Iced Tea Mix Lemon	6 oz	55	0	0
Lipton Iced Tea Sugar Free	8 oz	1	0	0
Lipton Iced Tea Sugar Free Peach	8 oz	5	0	0
Lipton Iced Tea Sugar Free Raspberry	8 oz	5	0	0
Lipton Iced Tea With Nutrasweet	8 oz	3	0	0
Lipton Iced Tea With Nutrasweet Decaffeinated	8 oz	3	0	0
Lipton Instant	6 oz	0	0	0
Lipton Instant Lemon	8 oz	3	0	0
Lipton Instant Raspberry	8 oz	3	0	0
Lipton Instant Tea Decaffeinated	6 oz	0	0	0
brewed tea	6 oz	2	0	0
instant, artifically sweetened, lemon flavored, as prep w/ water	8 oz	5	0	0
instant, sweetened, lemon flavor, as prep w/ water	9 oz	87	0	0
instant, unsweetened, lemon flavor, as prep w/ water	8 oz	4	0	0

FOOD	PORTION	CAL	VIT A	VIT C
instant, unsweetened, as prep w/ water	8 oz	2	0	0

TEMPEH
tempeh	½ cup	165	569	0

TOFU
Azumaya Green Label	3.5 oz	68	30	1
Azumaya Name Age Fried	3.5 oz	144	130	1
firm	½ cup	183	209	tr
firm	¼ block (3 oz)	118	134	tr
fresh, fried	1 piece (.5 oz)	35	0	0
koyadofu, dried/frozen	1 piece (.5 oz)	82	88	tr
okara	½ cup	47	0	0
regular	½ cup	94	105	tr
regular	¼ block (4 oz)	88	99	tr
YOGURT Stir Fruity Black Cherry	6 oz	141	196	2
Stir Fruity Blueberry	6 oz	140	43	5
Stir Fruity Orange	6 oz	143	34	5
Stir Fruity Strawberry	6 oz	140	34	3

TOMATILLO
fresh	1 (1.2 oz)	11	39	4
fresh, chopped	½ cup	21	75	8

TOMATO
CANNED Health Valley Sauce	1 cup	70	4916	tr
Health Valley Sauce Low Sodium	1 cup	70	4916	tr

FOOD	PORTION	CAL	VIT A	VIT C
Hunt's				
Crushed Angela Mia	4 oz	35	144	22
Crushed Italian	4 oz	40	133	20
Italian Pear Shaped	4 oz	20	75	12
Paste	2 oz	45	200	27
Paste Italian Style	2 oz	50	200	27
Paste No Salt Added	2 oz	45	190	28
Paste With Garlic	2 oz	50	200	27
Peeled Choice-Cut	4 oz	20	118	18
Puree	4 oz	45	160	27
Sauce	4 oz	30	100	15
Sauce Herb	4 oz	70	125	18
Sauce Italian	4 oz	60	125	20
Sauce Meatloaf Fixin's	4 oz	20	60	12
Sauce No Salt Added	4 oz	35	125	27
Sauce Special	4 oz	35	100	15
Sauce With Bits	4 oz	30	125	18
Sauce With Garlic	4 oz	70	175	24
Sauce With Mushrooms	4 oz	25	100	15
Stewed	4 oz	35	75	18
Stewed Italian	4 oz	40	133	20
Stewed No Salt Added	4 oz	35	75	18
Whole	4 oz	20	75	12
Whole Italian	4 oz	25	133	20
Whole No Salt Added	4 oz	20	75	18
S&W				
Aspic Supreme	½ cup	60	400	2
Diced in Rich Puree	½ cup	35	740	18
Italian Stewed Sliced	½ cup	35	500	15
Italian Style w/ Basil	½ cup	25	750	15
Mexican Style Stewed	½ cup	40	800	12

FOOD	PORTION	CAL	VIT A	VIT C
Paste	6 oz	150	4500	48
Peeled Ready Cut	½ cup	25	750	18
Puree	½ cup	60	750	21
Sauce	½ cup	40	750	6
Sauce Chunky	½ cup	45	750	15
Stewed Sliced	½ cup	35	500	15
Stewed 50% Salt Reduced	½ cup	35	750	12
Whole Diet	½ cup	25	750	18
Whole Peeled	½ cup	25	750	18
paste	¼ cup	110	3234	55
puree	1 cup	102	3402	88
puree w/o salt	1 cup	102	3402	88
red, whole	½ cup	24	725	18
sauce	½ cup	37	1195	16
sauce, spanish style	½ cup	40	1202	11
sauce w/ mushrooms	½ cup	42	1165	15
sauce w/ onion	½ cup	52	1038	16
stewed	½ cup	34	710	17
stewed w/ green chiles	½ cup	18	468	8
wedges in tomato juice	½ cup	34	757	19
DRIED				
sun dried	1 cup	140	472	21
sun dried	1 piece	5	17	1
sun dried, in oil	1 cup (4 oz)	235	1415	112
sun dried, in oil	1 piece (3 g)	6	39	3
FRESH				
cooked	½ cup	32	892	27
green	1	30	789	29
red	1 (4.5 oz)	26	766	24
red, chopped	1 cup	35	2039	32

FOOD	PORTION	CAL	VIT A	VIT C
JUICE				
Campbell	6 oz	40	750	16
Hunt's	6 oz	30	125	18
No Salt Added	6 oz	35	187	20
Libby's	6 oz	35	1000	24
S&W California	6 oz	35	1000	15
S&W Diet	½ cup	35	1000	15
beef broth & tomato	5½ oz	61	215	2
clam & tomato	1 can (5.5 oz)	77	357	7
tomato juice	½ cup	21	678	22
tomato juice	6 oz	32	1012	33
TAKE-OUT				
stewed	1 cup	80	673	18

TONGUE

pork, braised	3 oz	230	0	1

TREE FERN

chopped, cooked	½ cup	28	142	21

TROUT
(The vitamin A in trout comes from animal sources.)

FOOD	PORTION	CAL	VIT A	VIT C
FRESH				
baked	3 oz	162	54	tr
rainbow, cooked	3 oz	129	63	3

TUNA
(The vitamin A in tuna comes mostly from animal sources
or from added plant ingredients.)

CANNED				
light in water	1 can (5.8 oz)	192	92	0
light in water	3 oz	99	47	0

FOOD	PORTION	CAL	VIT A	VIT C

TUNA DISHES
(The vitamin A in tuna dishes comes from animal and plant sources.)

FOOD	PORTION	CAL	VIT A	VIT C
FROZEN				
Microwave Tuna Sandwich (Mrs. Paul's)	1	200	tr	tr
TAKE-OUT				
tuna salad	1 cup	383	199	5
tuna salad	3 oz	159	82	1
tuna salad submarine sandwich w/ lettuce & oil	1	584	188	4

TURKEY
(The vitamin A in turkey is from animal sources; in prepared dishes, some may come from plant sources.)

FOOD	PORTION	CAL	VIT A	VIT C
CANNED				
w/ broth	1 can (5 oz)	231	0	3
w/ broth	½ can (2.5 oz)	116	0	1
FRESH				
back w/ skin, roasted	½ back (9 oz)	637	0	0
breast w/ skin, roasted	4 oz	212	0	0
dark meat w/ skin, roasted	3.6 oz	230	0	0
dark meat w/o skin, roasted	1 cup (5 oz)	262	0	0
dark meat w/o skin, roasted	3 oz	170	0	0
ground, cooked	3 oz	188	0	0
leg w/ skin, roasted	1 (1.2 lbs)	1133	0	0
leg w/ skin, roasted	2.5 oz	147	0	0
light meat w/ skin, roasted	4.7 oz	268	0	0
light meat w/ skin, roasted	from ½ turkey (2.3 lbs)	2069	0	0
light meat w/o skin, roasted	4 oz	183	0	0
neck, simmered	1 (5.3 oz)	274	0	0
skin, roasted	1 oz	141	0	0

FOOD	PORTION	CAL	VIT A	VIT C
skin, roasted	from ½ turkey (9 oz)	1096	0	0
w/ skin, neck & giblets, roasted	½ turkey (8.8 lbs)	4123	4631	1
w/ skin, roasted	½ turkey (4 lbs)	3857	0	0
w/ skin, roasted	8.4 oz	498	0	0
w/o skin, roasted	1 cup (5 oz)	238	0	0
w/o skin, roasted	7.3 oz	354	0	0
wing w/ skin, roasted	1 (6.5 oz)	426	0	0
READY-TO-USE Carl Buddig	1 oz	50	0	0
Carl Buddig Turkey Ham	1 oz	40	0	0
breast	1 slice (.75 oz)	23	0	0
poultry salad sandwich spread	1 oz	238	39	0
poultry salad sandwich spread	1 tbsp	109	18	0
prebasted breast w/ skin, roasted	1 breast (3.8 lbs)	2175	0	0
prebasted breast w/ skin, roasted	½ breast (1.9 lbs)	1087	0	0
turkey loaf breast meat	1 pkg (6 oz)	187	0	0
turkey loaf breast meat	2 slices (1.5 oz)	47	0	0

TURNIPS

CANNED greens	½ cup	17	4196	18
FRESH cooked, mashed	½ cup (4.2 oz)	47	674	23
cubed, cooked	½ cup (3 oz)	33	477	17
greens, chopped, cooked	½ cup	15	3959	20
greens, raw, chopped	½ cup	7	2128	17
raw, cubed	½ cup (2.4 oz)	25	406	18

FOOD	PORTION	CAL	VIT A	VIT C
FROZEN				
greens, cooked	½ cup	24	6540	18

VEAL DISHES
(The vitamin A in veal dishes comes from animal sources or from plant sources like tomato sauce.)

TAKE-OUT				
parmigiana	4.2 oz	279	1204	15

VEGETABLES MIXED

CANNED				
Chop Suey Vegetables (La Choy)	½ cup	10	80	6
Garden Medley (Green Giant)	½ cup	40	1500	0
Garden Salad Marinated (S&W)	½ cup	60	9500	2
Mixed Vegetables Old Fashion Harvest Time (S&W)	½ cup	35	5500	5
Peas & Carrots Water Pack (S&W)	½ cup	35	4500	7
Sweet Peas & Diced Carrots (S&W)	½ cup	50	5000	6
Sweet Peas With Tiny Pearl Onions (S&W)	½ cup	60	200	6
mixed vegetables	½ cup	39	9551	4
peas & carrots	½ cup	48	7386	8
peas & carrots, low sodium	½ cup	48	7386	8
peas & onions	½ cup	30	96	2
succotash	½ cup	102	187	9
FROZEN				
Green Giant				
American Mixtures California	½ cup	25	7000	27
American Mixtures Heartland	½ cup	25	2250	33

FOOD	PORTION	CAL	VIT A	VIT C
Green Giant *(cont.)*				
American Mixtures New England	½ cup	70	4000	9
American Mixtures San Francisco	½ cup	25	200	27
American Mixtures Sante Fe	½ cup	70	500	15
American Mixtures Seattle	½ cup	25	5000	21
Breaded Medley (Ore Ida)	3 oz	160	2500	2
Broccoli, Cauliflower And Carrots In Butter Sauce (Green Giant)	½ cup	30	4000	21
Broccoli, Cauliflower And Carrots In Cheese Sauce (Green Giant)	½ cup	60	1500	12
Broccoli, Cauliflower And Carrots With Cheese Sauce (Birds Eye)	½ pkg	80	1250	21
California Florentine Blend (Big Valley)	3.5 oz	25	4000	36
Farm Fresh Broccoli Cauliflower And Carrots (Birds Eye)	¾ cup	35	9000	42
Farm Fresh Broccoli And Cauliflower (Birds Eye)	¾ cup	30	1500	90
Farm Fresh Broccoli, Carrots And Water Chestnuts (Birds Eye)	¾ cup	40	7500	36
Farm Fresh Broccoli, Cauliflower and Red Peppers (Birds Eye)	¾ cup	30	1750	90
Farm Fresh Broccoli, Corn And Red Peppers (Birds Eye)	⅔ cup	60	1750	36
Farm Fresh Broccoli, Green Beans, Pearl Onions and Red Peppers (Birds Eye)	¾ cup	35	1500	36

FOOD	PORTION	CAL	VIT A	VIT C
Farm Fresh Broccoli, Red Peppers, Onions And Mushrooms (Birds Eye)	¾ cup	30	2250	54
Farm Fresh Brussels Sprouts Cauliflower And Carrots (Birds Eye)	¾ cup	40	5500	54
Farm Fresh Cauliflower, Carrots And Snow Peas (Birds Eye)	⅔ cup	35	7500	30
Harvest Fresh Mixed Vegetables (Green Giant)	½ cup	40	4000	6
In Butter Sauce Broccoli, Cauliflower And Carrots (Birds Eye)	½ cup	40	4500	27
Internationals Austrian (Birds Eye)	3.3 oz	70	300	21
Internationals Bavarian (Birds Eye)	3.3 oz	90	1500	6
Internationals California (Birds Eye)	3.3 oz	90	2000	15
Internationals French Country (Birds Eye)	3.3 oz	70	1750	15
Internationals Japanese (Birds Eye)	3.3 oz	60	400	24
Internationals New England (Birds Eye)	3.3 oz	100	400	15
Internationals Italian (Birds Eye)	3.3 oz	80	400	24
Mandarin Vegetables (Budget Gourmet)	1 pkg.	160	4000	15
Mixed (Birds Eye)	½ cup	60	6500	9
Mixed (Green Giant)	½ cup	40	4000	5
Mixed Fancy (La Choy)	½ cup	12	20	9
Mixed In Butter Sauce (Green Giant)	½ cup	60	4000	4

FOOD	PORTION	CAL	VIT A	VIT C
New England Recipe Vegetables (Budget Gourmet)	1 pkg	230	750	15
One Serve Broccoli, Carrots & Rotini In Cheese Sauce (Green Giant)	1 pkg	120	9500	24
One Serve Broccoli, Cauliflower And Carrots (Green Giant)	1 pkg	25	2500	42
Peas & Cauliflower In Cream Sauce (Budget Gourmet)	1 pkg	150	1000	21
Peas And Potatoes With Cream Sauce (Birds Eye)	½ cup	100	200	6
Peas And Waterchestnuts Oriental (Budget Gourmet)	1 pkg	110	1500	9
Polybag (Birds Eye)	½ cup	60	6000	9
Spring Vegetables in Cheese Sauce (Budget Gourmet)	1 pkg	150	3000	36
Stew Vegetables (Ore Ida)	3 oz	50	4500	4
Valley Combinations Broccoli & Cauliflower (Green Giant)	½ cup	60	1250	21
mixed vegetables, cooked	½ cup	54	3892	3
peas & carrots, cooked	½ cup	38	6209	7
peas & onions, cooked	½ cup	40	313	6
succotash, cooked	½ cup	79	196	5
HOME RECIPE succotash	½ cup	111	282	8
JUICE Smucker's Vegetable Juice Hearty	8 oz	58	900	6
Smucker's Vegetable Juice Hot & Spicy	8 oz	58	1000	5
V8	6 oz	35	2250	20
V8 No Salt Added	6 oz	35	2500	20
V8 Spicy Hot	6 oz	35	2500	24

FOOD	PORTION	CAL	VIT A	VIT C
vegetable juice cocktail	½ cup	22	1416	34
vegetable juice cocktail	6 oz	34	2130	50
TAKE-OUT				
curry	1 serv (7.7 oz)	398	7845	26
pakoras	1 (2 oz)	108	390	3
ratatouille	8.8 oz	190	390	13
samosa	2 (4 oz)	519	170	4

VINEGAR

cider	1 tbsp	tr	0	0

WAFFLES

(The vitamin A in waffles comes from animal ingredients like milk and eggs or from plant sources like bran or blueberries.)

FOOD	PORTION	CAL	VIT A	VIT C
FROZEN				
Apple Cinnamon (Aunt Jemima)	2.5 oz	176	0	tr
Apple Cinnamon (Eggo)	1	130	500	0
Blueberry (Aunt Jemima)	2.5 oz	175	0	0
Blueberry (Eggo)	1	130	500	0
Blueberry Batter, as prep (Aunt Jemima)	3.6 oz	204	0	0
Buttermilk (Aunt Jemima)	2.5 oz	179	0	0
Buttermilk (Eggo)	1	130	500	0
Homestyle (Eggo)	1	130	500	0
Minis (Eggo)	4	90	500	0
Multi Bran (Nutri-Grain)	1	120	500	0
Nut And Honey (Eggo)	1	130	500	0
Oat Bran (Common Sense)	1	110	500	0
Oat Bran With Fruit And Nut (Common Sense)	1	120	500	0
Original (Aunt Jemima)	2.5 oz	173	0	0

FOOD	PORTION	CAL	VIT A	VIT C
Plain (Nutri-Grain)	1	120	500	0
Raisin And Bran (Nutri-Grain)	1	120	500	0
Special K (Kellogg's)	1	80	500	0
Wholegrain Wheat/Oat Bran (Aunt Jemima)	2.5 oz	154	0	0
buttermilk	1 4-in sq (1.2 oz)	88	448	0
plain	1 4-in sq (1.2 oz)	88	448	0
HOME RECIPE plain	1 (7-in diam)	218	140	tr
MIX plain, as prep	1 7-in diam (2.6 oz)	218	68	tr

WALNUTS

english, dried	1 oz	182	35	1
english, dried, chopped	1 cup	770	148	4

WATER CHESTNUTS

CANNED chinese, sliced	½ cup	35	3	1
FRESH sliced	½ cup	66	0	3

WATERCRESS

raw, chopped	½ cup	2	799	7

WATERMELON

cut up	1 cup	50	585	15
wedge	1⁄16	152	1762	47
SEEDS dried	1 cup	602	0	0

FOOD	PORTION	CAL	VIT A	VIT C
WHEAT GERM				
Kretschmer	¼ cup	103	33	0
Kretschmer Honey Crunch	¼ cup	105	0	0
WHIPPED TOPPINGS				
(The vitamin A in nondairy whipped toppings comes from plant sources.)				
cream, pressurized	1 cup	154	548	0
cream, pressurized	1 tbsp	8	27	0
nondairy powdered, as prep w/ whole milk	1 cup	151	289	1
nondairy powdered, as prep w/ whole milk	1 tbsp	8	14	tr
nondairy, pressurized	1 cup	184	331	0
nondairy, pressurized	1 tbsp	11	19	0
nondairy, frzn	1 tbsp	13	34	0
WHITE BEANS				
CANNED				
Goya Spanish Style	7.5 oz	130	844	2
white beans	1 cup	306	0	0
DRIED				
regular, cooked	1 cup	249	0	0
small, cooked	1 cup	253	0	0
WILD RICE				
cooked	½ cup	83	0	0
WINE				
red	3.5 oz	74	0	0
white	3.5 oz	70	0	0

FOOD	PORTION	CAL	VIT A	VIT C

WINGED BEANS

DRIED
| cooked | 1 cup | 252 | 0 | 0 |

YAM

CANNED
Bruce Cut	½ cup	139	6500	9
Bruce Mashed	½ cup	130	10000	9
Bruce Vacuum Pack	½ cup	122	7500	18
Bruce Whole	½ cup	139	6500	9
S&W Candied	½ cup	180	750	12
S&W Southern Whole in Extra Heavy Syrup	½ cup	139	6500	9

FRESH
| hawaii mountain yam, cooked | ½ cup | 59 | 0 | 0 |
| yam, cubed, cooked | ½ cup | 79 | 0 | 8 |

YAMBEAN

| cooked | ¾ cup | 38 | 19 | 14 |

YARDLONG BEANS

DRIED
| cooked | 1 cup | 202 | 27 | 1 |

YEAST

| brewer's dry | 1 tbsp | 25 | tr | tr |

YELLOW BEANS

DRIED
| cooked | 1 cup | 254 | 4 | 3 |

YELLOWTAIL
(The vitamin A in yellowtail comes from animal sources.)

FRESH
| baked | 3 oz | 159 | 88 | 2 |

FOOD	PORTION	CAL	VIT A	VIT C

YOGURT

(The vitamin A in yogurt comes from animal sources; fruit-flavored yogurts have a small amount from plant sources like blueberries.)

FOOD	PORTION	CAL	VIT A	VIT C
All Flavors (Cabot)	8 oz	220	100	1
Apple Crisp Lowfat (New Country)	6 oz	150	tr	tr
B! Lowfat French Style (Colombo)	6 oz	140	400	2
Banana Fruit On Bottom (Dannon)	8 oz	240	100	0
Blueberry (Dannon)	8 oz	200	100	0
Blueberry Supreme Lowfat (New Country)	6 oz	150	tr	tr
Blueberry Fruit On Bottom (Dannon)	4.4 oz	130	0	0
Blueberry Fruit On Bottom (Dannon)	8 oz	240	100	0
Blueberry Nonfat (Dannon)	6 oz	140	0	6
Blueberry Nonfat Light (Dannon)	4.4 oz	60	0	0
Blueberry Nonfat Light (Dannon)	8 oz	100	0	0
Boysenberry Fruit On Bottom (Dannon)	8 oz	240	100	0
Cherry Fruit On Bottom (Dannon)	4.4 oz	130	0	0
Cherry Fruit On Bottom (Dannon)	8 oz	240	100	0
Cherry Supreme Lowfat (New Country)	6 oz	150	tr	tr
Cherry Vanilla Nonfat Light (Dannon)	8 oz	100	0	0
Coffee Lowfat (Dannon)	8 oz	200	100	0

FOOD	PORTION	CAL	VIT A	VIT C
Dutch Apple Fruit On Bottom (Dannon)	8 oz	240	100	0
Exotic Fruit Fruit On Bottom (Dannon)	8 oz	240	100	0
French Vanilla Lowfat (New Country)	6 oz	150	tr	tr
Fruit Crunch Lowfat (New Country)	6 oz	150	tr	tr
Hawaiian Salad Lowfat (New Country)	6 oz	150	tr	tr
Lemon Lowfat (Dannon)	8 oz	200	100	0
Lemon Supreme Lowfat (New Country)	6 oz	150	tr	tr
Mixed Berries Fruit On Bottom (Dannon)	4.4 oz	130	0	0
Mixed Berries Fruit On Bottom (Dannon)	8 oz	240	100	0
Mixed Berries Lowfat (Dannon)	8 oz	240	100	0
Mixed Berries Lowfat (New Country)	6 oz	150	tr	tr
Orange Supreme Lowfat (New Country)	6 oz	150	tr	tr
Peach Fruit On Bottom (Dannon)	8 oz	240	100	0
Peach Lowfat Blended With Fruit (Dannon)	4.4 oz	130	0	0
Peach Nonfat (Dannon)	6 oz	140	0	6
Peach Nonfat Light (Dannon)	8 oz	100	0	0
Peaches 'n Cream Lowfat (New Country)	6 oz	150	tr	tr
Pina Colada Fruit On Bottom (Dannon)	8 oz	240	100	0
Plain (Cabot)	8 oz	140	200	2
Plain Lowfat (Dannon)	8 oz	140	100	0

FOOD	PORTION	CAL	VIT A	VIT C
Plain Nonfat (Dannon)	8 oz	110	0	0
Raspberry Supreme Lowfat (New Country)	6 oz	150	tr	tr
Raspberry Fruit On Bottom (Dannon)	4.4 oz	120	0	0
Raspberry Fruit On Bottom (Dannon)	8 oz	240	100	0
Raspberry Lowfat Blended With Fruit (Dannon)	4.4 oz	130	0	0
Raspberry Nonfat (Dannon)	6 oz	140	0	0
Raspberry Nonfat (Dannon)	8 oz	200	100	0
Raspberry Nonfat Light (Dannon)	8 oz	100	0	0
Strawberry Banana Fruit On Bottom (Dannon)	4.4 oz	130	0	0
Strawberry Banana Lowfat (New Country)	6 oz	150	tr	tr
Strawberry Banana Lowfat Blended With Fruit (Dannon)	4.4 oz	130	0	0
Strawberry Banana Nonfat Light (Dannon)	8 oz	100	0	0
Strawberry Lowfat (Dannon)	8 oz	200	100	0
Strawberry Lowfat Blended With Fruit (Dannon)	4.4 oz	130	0	0
Strawberry Nonfat (Dannon)	6 oz	140	0	6
Strawberry Nonfat Light (Dannon)	4.4 oz	60	0	0
Strawberry Nonfat Light (Dannon)	8 oz	100	0	0
Strawberry Supreme Lowfat (New Country)	6 oz	150	tr	tr
Strawberry Fruit Cup Lowfat (New Country)	6 oz	150	tr	tr
Strawberry Fruit Cup Nonfat Light (Dannon)	8 oz	100	0	0

FOOD	PORTION	CAL	VIT A	VIT C
Strawberry Fruit On Bottom (Dannon)	4.4 oz	130	0	0
Strawberry Fruit On Bottom (Dannon)	8 oz	240	100	0
Vanilla Lowfat (Dannon)	8 oz	200	100	0
Vanilla Nonfat Light (Dannon)	8 oz	100	0	0
coffee, lowfat	8 oz	194	123	2
fruit, lowfat	4 oz	113	56	1
fruit, lowfat	8 oz	225	111	1
plain	8 oz	139	279	1
plain, lowfat	8 oz	144	150	2
plain, nonfat	8 oz	127	16	2
vanilla, lowfat	8 oz	194	123	2

YOGURT FROZEN

FOOD	PORTION	CAL	VIT A	VIT C
Strawberry (Borden)	½ cup	100	0	0
Strawberry (Meadow Gold)	½ cup	100	0	0
Strawberry Nonfat (Dannon)	6 oz	140	0	6

ZUCCHINI

FOOD	PORTION	CAL	VIT A	VIT C
CANNED				
Italian Style (S&W)	½ cup	45	1250	6
Italian Style	½ cup	33	615	3
FRESH				
baby, raw	1 (.5 oz)	3	78	6
raw, slices	½ cup	9	221	6
sliced, cooked	½ cup	14	216	4
FROZEN				
Big Valley	3.5 oz	12	300	7
Breaded Zucchini (Ore Ida)	3 oz	150	200	2
cooked	½ cup	19	483	4

PART II

Vitamin A and
Vitamin C Values
for Restaurants and Fast-Food Chains

The following listing does not include all menu items, just those that contribute the antioxidant vitamins A and C.

Vitamin A content in the following listing may be from either animal or plant sources.

ALL VITAMIN A VALUES ARE GIVEN IN INTERNATIONAL UNITS (IU).
ALL VITAMIN C VALUES ARE GIVEN IN MILLIGRAMS (MG).

FOOD	PORTION	CAL	VIT A	VIT C

ARBY'S

BAKED SELECTIONS

FOOD	PORTION	CAL	VIT A	VIT C
Turnover, Apple	1	303	100	1

BEVERAGES

Milk Lo Fat 2%	8 oz	121	500	2

BREAKFAST SELECTIONS

Platter, Bacon	1	860	400	4
Platter, Egg	1	460	400	4
Platter, Ham	1	518	400	4
Platter, Sausage	1	640	400	4

MAIN MENU SELECTIONS

Baked Potato, Broccoli 'N Cheddar	1	417	300	45
Baked Potato, Deluxe	1	621	500	33
Baked Potato, Mushroom & Cheese	1	515	1750	33
Baked Potato, With Butter/ Margarine And Sour Cream	1	463	200	33
Ketchup	0.5 oz	16	250	1
Philly Beef 'N Swiss Sandwich	1	498	300	2
Roast Beef Sandwich, Super	1	529	300	1
Turkey Deluxe Sandwich	1	399	300	5

SALAD DRESSINGS

Honey French Dressing	2 oz	322	400	1

SALADS AND SALAD BARS

Cashew Chicken Salad	1	590	1000	5
Chef Salad	1	210	1500	6
Garden Salad	1	149	1500	6

SOUPS

Beef With Vegetables & Barley	8 oz	96	1500	5
Boston Clam Chowder	8 oz	207	500	4
Cream of Broccoli	8 oz	180	500	9
French Onion	8 oz	67	100	2

FOOD	PORTION	CAL	VIT A	VIT C
Lumberjack Mixed Vegetable	8 oz	89	2500	9
Pilgrim's Corn Chowder	5 oz	193	1750	4
Split Pea With Ham	8 oz	200	1500	1
Tomato Florentine	8 oz	244	1000	12
Wisconsin Cheese	8 oz	287	300	2

AU BON PAIN

BREAD AND ROLLS

Alpine Roll	1	220	0	0
Baguette Loaf	1	810	0	0
Cheese Loaf	1	1670	450	0
Four Grain Loaf	1	1420	22	0
French Roll	1	320	0	0
Hearth Roll	1	250	6	0
Hearth Sandwich Roll	1	370	9	0
Onion Herb Loaf	1	1430	0	0
Parisienne Loaf	1	1490	0	0
Petit Pain Roll	1	220	0	0
Sandwich Croissant	1	300	495	0
Soft Roll	1	310	156	0

COOKIES

Chocolate Chip	1	280	419	0
Chocolate Chunk Pecan	1	290	386	0
Oatmeal Raisin	1	250	415	0
Peanut Butter	1	290	323	0
White Chocolate Chunk Pecan	1	300	430	0

CROISSANTS

Almond	1	420	750	0
Apple	1	250	390	2
Blueberry Cheese	1	380	770	0
Chocolate	1	400	510	0

FOOD	PORTION	CAL	VIT A	VIT C
Chocolate Hazelnut	1	480	510	0
Cinnamon Raisin	1	390	460	1
Coconut Pecan	1	440	600	0
Ham & Cheese	1	370	720	0
Plain	1	220	360	0
Raspberry Cheese	1	400	770	0
Spinach & Cheese	1	290	2780	4
Strawberry Cheese	1	400	770	0
Sweet Cheese	1	420	909	0
Turkey & Cheddar	1	410	750	0
Turkey & Havarti	1	410	720	0
MUFFINS Blueberry	1	390	490	0
Bran	1	390	160	1
Carrot	1	450	6110	3
Corn	1	460	73	0
Cranberry Walnut	1	350	82	3
Oat Bran Apple	1	400	17	2
Pumpkin	1	410	9520	3
Whole Grain	1	440	82	0
SALADS AND SALAD BARS Chicken, Cracked Pepper	1	100	6050	47
Chicken, Grilled	1	110	6050	46
Garden, Large	1	40	6050	46
Garden, Small	1	20	3090	24
Shrimp	1	102	6250	47
SANDWICHES AND FILLINGS Boursin	1 serv	290	1200	0
Swiss	1 serv	330	730	0
SOUPS Beef Barley	1 bowl	125	150	0

FOOD	PORTION	CAL	VIT A	VIT C
Beef Barley	1 cup	80	100	0
Chicken Noodle	1 bowl	125	155	0
Chicken Noodle	1 cup	80	100	0
Clam Chowder	1 bowl	390	300	2
Clam Chowder	1 cup	270	200	1
Cream of Broccoli	1 bowl	380	1000	9
Cream of Broccoli	1 cup	250	750	6
Garden Vegetarian	1 bowl	70	2000	9
Garden Vegetarian	1 cup	50	1250	6
Minestrone	1 bowl	190	1000	9
Minestrone	1 cup	120	750	6
Split Pea	1 bowl	380	1500	4
Split Pea	1 cup	250	1000	2
Tomato Florentine	1 bowl	120	2750	18
Tomato Florentine	1 cup	90	1750	12
Vegetarian Chili	1 bowl	280	3250	24
Vegetarian Chili	1 cup	180	2000	15

BURGER KING

BAKED SELECTIONS

Cherry Pie	1	360	300	6

BEVERAGES

Milk 2%	1	121	500	2
Orange Juice	1	82	150	71
Shake Chocolate	1 med	284	350	2

BREAKFAST SELECTIONS

Hash Browns	1	213	600	5

MAIN MENU SELECTIONS

BK Broiler	1	280	100	4
Bacon Double Cheeseburger Deluxe	1	530	500	2
Cheeseburger	1	300	300	2

FOOD	PORTION	CAL	VIT A	VIT C
Dipping Sauce Barbecue	1 oz	36	150	2
Double Cheeseburger	1	450	500	2
Double Whopper	1	800	400	12
Hamburger	1	260	100	2
Ketchup	0.5 oz	17	250	5
Tomato	1 oz	6	200	5
Whopper	1	570	400	12
Whopper, Double With Cheese	1	890	1000	12
Whopper Jr.	1	300	200	5
Whopper Jr. With Cheese	1	350	400	5
Whopper With Cheese	1	660	1000	12
SALADS AND SALAD BARS Chef Salad w/o Dressing	1	178	4750	15
Chunky Chicken Salad w/o Dressing	1	142	4600	20
Garden Salad w/o Dressing	1	95	5000	35
Side Salad	1	25	4400	12

CARL'S JR.

BEVERAGES Milk 2%	10 oz	180	300	2
Orange Juice	1 sm	90	200	72
MAIN MENU SELECTIONS Cheeseburger, Double Western w/ Bacon	1	1030	2000	6
Cheeseburger, Western w/ Bacon	1	730	1250	4
Chicken Club Charbroiler	1	570	1250	1
Chicken Sante Fe Sandwich	1	540	300	6
Country Fried Steak Sandwich	1	720	750	1
Hamburger	1	220	500	1
Hamburger, Famous Star	1	610	1500	4

FOOD	PORTION	CAL	VIT A	VIT C
Hamburger, Old Time Star	1	460	1000	4
Hamburger, Super Star	1	820	2000	6
Potato, Bacon & Cheese	1	730	1250	2
Potato, Broccoli & Cheese	1	590	2500	2
Potato, Fiesta	1	720	2000	2
Potato, Sour Cream & Chives	1	470	750	1
Potato w/ Cheese	1	690	1500	2
Roast Beef Club	1	620	1250	2
Roast Beef Deluxe Sandwich	1	540	1500	6
SALADS AND SALAD BARS				
Salad-To-Go, Chicken	1	200	250	5
Salad-To-Go, Garden	1 sm	50	150	1

CARVEL

FOOD	PORTION	CAL	VIT A	VIT C
Lo-Yo Vanilla Frozen Yogurt (Carvel)	1 oz	34	100	tr

DAIRY QUEEN/BRAZIER

FOOD	PORTION	CAL	VIT A	VIT C
FOOD SELECTION				
DQ Homestyle Ultimate Burger	1	700	1000	9
Garden Salad w/o dressing	1	200	3000	21
Grilled Chicken Fillet Sandwich	1	300	100	2
Side Salad w/o dressing	1	25	2500	15
Thousand Island Dressing	2 oz	225	200	2
Tomato	0.5 oz	3	100	2
ICE CREAM				
Blizzard, Strawberry	1 reg	740	400	24
Blizzard, Strawberry	1 sm	500	300	15
Waffle Cone Sundae, Strawberry	1	350	200	6

FOOD	PORTION	CAL	VIT A	VIT C
EL POLLO LOCO				
Beans	3.5 oz	110	0	0
Chicken	2 pieces	310	0	0
Coleslaw	2.8 oz	80	0	15
Combo Meal	1	720	100	24
Corn	3.3 oz	110	400	6
Potato Salad	4.3 oz	140	100	9
Salsa	1.8 oz	10	0	9
Tortillas, Corn	3.3 oz	210	0	0
Tortillas, Flour	3.3 oz	280	0	0
GODFATHER'S PIZZA				
Golden Crust Cheese	1/10 lg	261	450	6
Golden Crust Cheese	1/6 sm	213	400	5
Golden Crust Cheese	1/8 med	229	400	5
Golden Crust Combo	1/10 lg	322	500	7
Golden Crust Combo	1/6 sm	273	400	6
Golden Crust Combo	1/8 med	283	400	6
Original Crust Cheese	1/10 lg	271	550	6
Original Crust Cheese	1/4 mini	138	250	1
Original Crust Cheese	1/6 sm	239	500	5
Original Crust Cheese	1/8 med	242	450	5
Original Crust Combo	1/10 lg	332	550	7
Original Crust Combo	1/4 mini	164	250	3
Original Crust Combo	1/6 sm	299	500	6
Original Crust Combo	1/8 med	318	550	6
HAAGEN-DAZS				
Orange & Cream Pop	1	130	300	6

FOOD	PORTION	CAL	VIT A	VIT C

JACK IN THE BOX

BEVERAGES

Lowfat Milk 2%	8 oz	122	500	2
Orange Juice	6 oz	80	400	96

BREAKFAST SELECTIONS

Pancake Platter	1	612	400	6
Scrambled Egg Platter	1	559	700	10
Sourdough Breakfast Sandwich	1	381	700	7

MAIN MENU SELECTIONS

Bacon Bacon Cheeseburger	1	705	350	8
Chicken & Mushroom Sandwich	1	438	450	2
Chicken Supreme	1	641	400	6
Old Fashioned Patty Melt	1	713	550	4

SALADS AND SALAD BARS

Chef Salad	1	325	3650	28
Taco Salad	1	503	1350	9

KENTUCKY FRIED CHICKEN

SIDE DISHES

Corn-on-the-Cob	1 ear (2.6 oz)	90	150	1

LITTLE CAESARS PIZZA

MAIN MENU SELECTIONS

Antipasto Salad	1 sm	96	500	12
Crazy Bread	1 piece	98	0	0
Crazy Sauce	1 serv	63	1000	18
Greek Salad	1 sm	85	750	12
Ham & Cheese Sandwich	1	552	500	15
Italian Sandwich	1	615	500	21
Tossed Salad	1 sm	37	400	9
Tuna Sandwich	1	610	500	60

FOOD	PORTION	CAL	VIT A	VIT C
Turkey Sandwich	1	450	100	12
Veggie Sandwich	1	784	2000	21
PIZZA Baby Pan! Pan!	1 order	525	1250	18
Cheese & Pepperoni, Round, Large	1 slice	185	400	6
Cheese & Pepperoni, Round, Medium	1 slice	168	400	6
Cheese & Pepperoni, Round, Small	1 slice	151	300	5
Cheese & Pepperoni, Square, Large	1 slice	204	500	5
Cheese & Pepperoni, Square, Medium	1 slice	201	500	5
Cheese & Pepperoni, Square, Small	1 slice	204	500	5
Cheese, Round, Large	1 slice	169	400	6
Cheese, Round, Medium	1 slice	154	500	6
Cheese, Round, Small	1 slice	138	300	5
Cheese, Square, Large	1 slice	188	500	5
Cheese, Square, Medium	1 slice	185	500	5
Cheese, Square, Small	1 slice	188	500	5
Slice! Slice!	1 order	756	1500	24

LONG JOHN SILVER'S

FOOD	PORTION	CAL	VIT A	VIT C
BAKED SELECTIONS Cherry Pie	1 slice	360	400	9
MAIN MENU SELECTIONS Chicken	17.3 oz	620	300	4
Chicken Planks, 3 Pieces w/ Fryes & Slaw	14.1 oz	860	200	18
Chicken Planks, 4 Pieces w/ Fryes & Slaw	16 oz	990	200	18
Clams w/ Fryes & Slaw	12.7 oz	910	200	15

FOOD	PORTION	CAL	VIT A	VIT C
Corn Cobbette	1 piece	140	300	9
Fish & Chicken w/ Fryes & Slaw	15.2 oz	930	200	18
Fish & More, 2 Pieces	14 oz	860	200	15
Fish & More, 3 Pieces w/ Fryes & Slaw	17.5 oz	1070	200	18
Fish Light Portion w/ Lemon Crumb, 2 Pieces	10.3 oz	320	1750	6
Fish Light Portion w/ Paprika, 2 Pieces	10 oz	300	1750	6
Fish w/ Lemon Crumb, 3 Pieces	18.4 oz	640	2500	4
Fish w/ Paprika, 3 Pieces	18.2 oz	610	2250	4
Fish w/ Scampi Sauce, 3 Pieces	18.6 oz	660	2250	4
Long John's Homestyle Fish, 3 Pieces w/ Fryes & Slaw	13.1 oz	830	500	15
Long John's Homestyle Fish, 4 Pieces w/ Fryes & Slaw	14.8 oz	960	750	15
Ocean Chef Salad	8.2 oz	234	3500	21
Seafood Salad	9.8 oz	230	3000	18
Shrimp Scampi	10.6 oz	610	400	4

McDONALD'S

FOOD	PORTION	CAL	VIT A	VIT C
BEVERAGES				
Milk 1%	8 oz	110	500	2
BREAKFAST SELECTIONS				
Breakfast Burrito	1	280	500	6
Cheerios	¾ cup	80	750	9
Wheaties	¾ cup	90	1000	12
ICE CREAM				
Sundae, Lowfat Frozen Yogurt, Strawberry	1 (6oz)	210	200	1
MAIN MENU SELECTIONS				
Big Mac	1	500	300	1

FOOD	PORTION	CAL	VIT A	VIT C
Cheeseburger	1	305	400	2
Chicken Fajita	1	185	100	5
Hamburger	1	255	200	2
McChicken	1	415	100	2
McLean Deluxe	1	320	500	6
McLean Deluxe w/ Cheese	1	370	750	6
Quarter Pounder	1	410	200	4
Quarter Pounder w/ Cheese	1	510	750	4
SALADS AND SALAD BARS Chef Salad	1 serv	170	5000	21
Chunky Chicken Salad	1 serv	150	8500	2
Garden Salad	1	50	4500	21
Side Salad	1 serv	30	4000	12
SAUCES McNuggets Sauce, Barbeque	1.12 fl oz	50	200	2

PIZZA HUT

FOOD	PORTION	CAL	VIT A	VIT C
Cheese Hand-Tossed Medium	2 slices	518	500	10
Cheese Pan Medium	2 slices	492	450	8
Pepperoni Hand-Tossed Medium	2 slices	500	500	7
Pepperoni Pan Medium	2 slices	540	500	8
Pepperoni Personal Pan	1 Pie	675	600	10
Pepperoni Thin 'n Crispy Medium	2 slices	413	350	6
Super Supreme Hand-Tossed Medium	2 slices	556	550	12
Super Supreme Pan Medium	2 slices	563	600	11
Supreme Hand-Tossed Medium	2 slices	540	550	12
Supreme Pan Medium	2 slices	589	600	10
Supreme Personal Pan	1 pie	647	600	11

FOOD	PORTION	CAL	VIT A	VIT C
Super Supreme	2 slices	463	500	8
Supreme	2 slices	459	500	10
Thin 'N Crispy Medium Cheese	2 slices	398	350	5

T.J. CINNAMONS

FOOD	PORTION	CAL	VIT A	VIT C
Doughnuts, Cake	2	454	100	0
Doughnuts, Raised	2	352	60	0
Mini-Cinn, Plain	1	75	225	tr
Mini-Cinn With Icing	1	80	225	tr
Original Gourmet Cinnamon Roll, Plain	1	630	1470	1
Original Gourmet Cinnamon Roll With Icing	1	686	1470	1
Petite Cinnamon Roll, Plain	1	185	440	tr
Petite Cinnamon Roll With Icing	1	202	440	tr
Sticky Bun Cinnamon, Pecan	1	607	1110	tr
Sticky Bun Petite, Cinnamon Pecan	1	255	445	tr
Triple Chocolate Classic Roll, Plain	1	412	1100	tr
Triple Chocolate Classic Roll With Icing	1	462	1260	tr

TACO BELL

FOOD	PORTION	CAL	VIT A	VIT C
Burrito, Bean	1	447	350	53
Burrito, Beef	1	493	500	2
Burrito, Chicken	1	334	450	11
Burrito, Combo	1	407	450	27
Burrito, Fiesta Bean	1	226	250	43
Burrito, Supreme	1	503	900	26
Enchirito	1	382	950	28

FOOD	PORTION	CAL	VIT A	VIT C
Guacamole	⅔ oz	34	100	3
Jalapeno Peppers	3.5 oz	20	250	2
MexiMelt, Beef	1	266	800	2
MexiMelt, Chicken	1	257	500	2
Mexican Pizza	1	575	1000	31
Nacho Cheese Sauce	2 oz	105	150	1
Nachos	1	346	550	2
Nachos, Bellgrande	1	649	1150	58
Nachos Supreme	1	367	700	30
Pico De Gallo	1 oz	8	250	2
Pintos 'N Cheese	1	190	450	52
Red Sauce	1 oz	10	250	1
Taco	1	183	350	1
Taco, Bellgrande	1	335	850	5
Taco, Fiesta	1	127	250	tr
Taco Salad	1	905	1650	75
Taco Salad w/o Shell	1	484	1650	74
Taco, Soft	1	225	200	1
Taco, Soft, Chicken	1	213	200	3
Taco, Soft, Supreme	1	272	450	3
Taco, Soft, Fiesta	1	147	150	tr
Taco, Soft, Steak	1	218	150	1
Taco Supreme	1	230	550	3
Tostada	1	243	650	45
Tostada, Fiesta	1	167	400	27

TACO JOHN'S

FOOD	PORTION	CAL	VIT A	VIT C
Bean Burrito	1	197	750	1
Beef Burrito	1	303	450	1
Chicken Burrito w/ Green Chili	1	344	3500	12

FOOD	PORTION	CAL	VIT A	VIT C
Chicken Super Taco Salad w/ Dressing	1	507	5000	17
Chicken Super Taco Salad w/o Dressing	1	377	5000	17
Chimichanga	1	464	4300	8
Chimichanga w/ Chicken	1	441	4150	8
Combo Burrito	1	250	600	1
Nachos	1 serv	468	900	3
Smothered Burrito w/ Green Chili	1	367	3650	12
Smothered Burrito w/ Texas Chili	1	455	3950	12
Softshell	1	224	1500	5
Softshell w/ Chicken	1	180	1500	5
Super Burrito	1	389	2100	5
Super Burrito w/ Chicken	1	366	1950	5
Super Nachos	1 serv	669	3100	8
Super Taco Bravo	1	361	2200	5
Super Taco Salad w/ 2 oz Dressing	1	558	5000	17
Super Taco Salad w/o Dressing	1	428	5000	17
Taco	1	178	1450	5
Taco Bravo	1	319	1800	5
Taco Burger	1	281	1300	5
Taco Salad w/ 2 oz Dressing	1	359	3000	10
Taco Salad w/o Dressing	1	228	3000	10

WENDY'S

BEVERAGES

Chocolate Milk	8 oz	160	750	2

CHILDREN'S MENU SELECTIONS

Kid's Meal Cheeseburger	1	300	100	1

FOOD	PORTION	CAL	VIT A	VIT C
Kid's Meal Hamburger	1	260	100	1
MAIN MENU SELECTIONS				
Big Classic	1	570	500	12
Chicken Sandwich	1	440	100	5
Chili	9 oz	220	750	9
Country Fried Steak Sandwich	1	440	100	1
Fish Fillet Sandwich	1	460	100	1
Grilled Chicken Sandwich	1	340	100	5
Hot Stuffed Potato, Bacon & Cheese	1	520	500	36
Hot Stuffed Potato, Broccoli & Cheese	1	400	700	36
Hot Stuffed Potato, Cheese	1	420	500	30
Hot Stuffed Potato, Chili & Cheese	1	500	750	36
Hot Stuffed Potato, Sour Cream & Chives	1	500	2500	45
Jr. Bacon Cheeseburger	1	430	100	9
Jr. Cheeseburger	1	310	100	2
Jr. Hamburger	1	260	100	2
Jr. Swiss Deluxe	1	360	200	6
Ketchup	1 tbsp	17	200	2
Single With Everything	1	420	250	9
SALADS AND SALAD BARS				
Broccoli	½ cup	12	300	39
Cantaloupe	2 oz	20	1000	18
Carrots	¼ cup	12	4000	2
Chef Salad	1	130	5000	36
Chives	1 oz	71	9750	188
Cole Slaw	2 oz	70	200	15
Garden Salad	1	70	5500	42
Green Peas	1 oz	21	200	5

FOOD	PORTION	CAL	VIT A	VIT C
Green Peppers	¼ cup	10	100	36
Lettuce, Iceberg	1 cup	8	100	2
Lettuce, Romaine	1 cup	9	750	12
Pasta Medley	2 oz	60	300	9
Peaches	2 pieces	31	400	1
Taco Salad	1	530	1500	24
Tomatoes	1 oz	6	100	6
Watermelon	2 oz	18	100	6
SAUCES Picante Sauce	2 oz	18	500	18
Spaghetti Meat Sauce	2 oz	60	200	2
Taco Sauce	1 oz	16	200	1

PART III

Vitamin E Values for
Brand-Name and Generic Foods

ALL VITAMIN E VALUES ARE GIVEN IN INTERNATIONAL
UNITS (IU).

FOOD	PORTION	CAL	VIT E

ALMONDS

FOOD	PORTION	CAL	VIT E
dried, blanched	1 oz	166	6
dried, unblanched	1 oz	167	7
oil roasted, blanched	1 oz	174	2
oil roasted, blanched, salted	1 oz	174	2
toasted, unblanched	1 oz	167	14

AMARANTH

FOOD	PORTION	CAL	VIT E
Amaranth Cereal With Bananas (Health Valley)	½ cup (1 oz)	110	2
Amaranth Crunch With Raisins (Health Valley)	¼ cup (1 oz)	110	tr
Amaranth Flakes 100% Organic (Health Valley)	½ cup (1 oz)	90	1
Fast Menu Amaranth With Garden Vegetables (Health Valley)	7.5 oz	140	1

ASPARAGUS

FOOD	PORTION	CAL	VIT E
FRESH			
raw	½ cup	16	1
raw	4 spears	14	1

BARLEY

FOOD	PORTION	CAL	VIT E
Quaker Medium Pearled	¼ cup	172	0
Quaker Quick Pearled	¼ cup	172	0
Scotch Medium Pearled	¼ cup	172	0
Scotch Quick Pearled	¼ cup	172	0
pearled, uncooked	½ cup	352	tr

BEANS

FOOD	PORTION	CAL	VIT E
CANNED			
Boston Baked (Health Valley)	7.5 oz	190	1
Boston Baked No Salt Added (Health Valley)	7.5 oz	190	1

FOOD	PORTION	CAL	VIT E
Vegetarian Beans With Miso (Health Valley)	7.5 oz	180	1
TAKE-OUT			
refried beans	½ cup	43	1
three bean salad	¾ cup	230	tr

BEEF DISHES

CANNED			
Beef Stew (Wolf Brand)	1 cup	179	2
TAKE-OUT			
Stroganoff	¾ cup	260	tr

BISCUIT

MIX			
Buttermilk Biscuit Mix, not prep (Health Valley)	1 oz	100	tr

BLACK BEANS

CANNED			
Health Valley Fast Menu Organic Black Beans With Tofu Wieners	7.5 oz	150	1

BLINTZE

TAKE-OUT			
cheese	2	186	tr

BRAN

Fast Menu Oat Bran Pilaf With Garden Vegetables (Health Valley)	7.5 oz	210	9
Oat Bran (Mother's)	⅓ cup	92	tr
Quaker Unprocessed Bran	2 tbsp	8	tr
Toasted Wheat Bran (Kretschmer)	⅓ cup	57	1
Wheat dry	½ cup	65	tr

FOOD	PORTION	CAL	VIT E

BRAZIL NUTS

| dried, unblanched | 1 oz | 186 | 2 |

BREAD

TAKE-OUT

| cornstick | 1 (1.3 oz) | 101 | tr |

BREAKFAST DRINKS

Pillsbury

Instant Breakfast Chocolate Malt, as prep w/ whole milk	1 serv	290	8
Instant Breakfast Chocolate, as prep w/ whole milk	1 serv	290	8
Instant Breakfast Strawberry, as prep w/ whole milk	1 serv	290	8
Instant Breakfast Vanilla, as prep w/ whole milk	1 serv	300	8

BROCCOLI

FRESH

| raw, chopped | ½ cup | 12 | tr |

BRUSSELS SPROUTS

cooked	1 sprout	8	tr
cooked	½ cup	30	1
raw	1 sprout	8	tr
raw	½ cup	19	tr

CABBAGE

chinese pe-tsai, raw, shredded	1 cup	12	tr
danish, raw, shredded	½ cup (1.2 oz)	9	1
green, raw	1 head (2 lbs)	228	15
green, raw, shredded	½ cup (1.2 oz)	9	tr

FOOD	PORTION	CAL	VIT E
TAKE-OUT			
stuffed cabbage	1 (6 oz)	373	tr
CAKE			
baklava	1 oz	126	tr
strudel	1 piece (4.1 oz)	272	1
CARROTS			
FRESH			
raw	1 (2.5 oz)	31	tr
raw, shredded	½ cup	24	tr
slices, cooked	½ cup	35	tr
CASHEWS			
dry roasted	1 oz	163	tr
dry roasted, salted	1 oz	163	tr
CAULIFLOWER			
FRESH			
flowerets, raw	3 (2 oz)	14	tr
raw	½ cup (1.8 oz)	13	tr
CELERY			
raw	1 stalk (1.3 oz)	6	tr
raw, diced	½ cup	10	tr
CEREAL			
COOKED			
Enriched White Hominy Grits Quick (Quaker)	3 tbsp	101	0
Enriched White Hominy Grits Regular (Aunt Jemima)	3 tbsp	101	0
Enriched Yellow Hominy Quick Grits (Quaker)	3 tbsp	101	0

FOOD	PORTION	CAL	VIT E
Instant Grits White Hominy (Quaker)	1 pkg	79	0
Instant Grits With Imitation Bacon Bits (Quaker)	1 pkg	101	0
Instant Grits With Imitation Ham Bits (Quaker)	1 pkg	99	0
Instant Grits With Real Cheddar Cheese (Quaker)	1 pkg	104	0
Oat Bran (Quaker)	⅓ cup	92	tr
Oat Bran Natural Apples & Cinnamon (Health Valley)	¼ cup (1 oz)	100	tr
Oat Bran Natural Raisins & Sprice (Health Valley)	¼ cup	100	tr
Quaker			
Oatmeal Instant Apples & Cinnamon	1 pkg	118	tr
Oatmeal Instant Extra Fortified Apples & Spice	1 pkg	133	30
Oatmeal Instant Extra Fortified Raisins & Cinnamon	1 pkg	129	30
Oatmeal Instant Extra Fortified Regular	1 pkg	95	30
Oatmeal Instant Maple & Brown Sugar	1 pkg	152	tr
Oatmeal Instant Peaches & Cream Quaker	1 pkg	129	tr
Oatmeal Instant Raisin & Spice	1 pkg	149	tr
Oatmeal Instant Raisin, Dates & Walnuts	1 pkg	141	tr
Oatmeal Instant Regular	1 pkg	94	tr
Oatmeal Instant Strawberries & Cream Flavors	1 pkg	129	tr
Oats Old Fashion	⅔ cup	99	tr
Oats Quick	⅔ cup	99	tr
Whole Wheat Hot Natural Cereal	⅔ cup	92	tr

FOOD	PORTION	CAL	VIT E
farina, not prep	1 tbsp	40	tr
oatmeal, not prep	1 cup	311	2
READY-TO-EAT			
100% Natural Bran With Apples & Cinnamon (Health Valley)	¼ cup (1 oz)	100	0
Body Buddies Natural Fruit (General Mills)	1 cup (1 oz)	110	8
Bran Cereal With Dates 100% Organic (Health Valley)	¼ cup (1 oz)	100	0
Bran Cereal With Raisins 100% Organic (Health Valley)	¼ cup (1 oz)	100	0
Crunchy Bran (Quaker)	⅔ cup	89	1
Healthy Valley			
Fiber 7 Flakes With Raisins 100% Organic	½ cup (1 oz)	90	0
Fruit & Fitness	1 cup (2 oz)	220	2
Fruit Lites Corn	½ cup (0.5 oz)	45	1
Fruit Lites Wheat	½ cup (0.5 oz)	45	1
Fruit Lites Rice	½ cup (.5 oz)	45	1
Healthy Crunch Almond Date	¼ cup (1 oz)	110	tr
Healthy Crunch Apple Cinnamon	¼ cup (1 oz)	110	tr
Healthy O's 100% Organic	¾ cup (1 oz)	90	4

CHEESE

NATURAL			
Emmentaler	3.5 oz	403	tr
Quark 20% fat	3.5 oz	116	tr
Quark 40% fat	3.5 oz	167	tr
Quark made w/ skim milk	3.5 oz	78	tr

CHEESE DISHES

TAKE-OUT			
fondue	½ cup	303	0

FOOD	PORTION	CAL	VIT E

CHICKEN DISHES

chicken cacciatore	¾ cup	394	8
chicken & dumplings	¾ cup	256	tr

CHILI

CANNED
Health Valley

Mild Vegetarian With Beans	5 oz	160	5
Mild Vegetarian With Beans No Salt Added	5 oz	160	5
Mild Vegetarian With Lentils	5 oz	140	12
Mild Vegetarian With Lentils No Salt Added	5 oz	140	12
Spicy Vegetarian With Beans	5 oz	160	2
Wolf Brand Chili-Mac	7.5 oz	317	2
Wolf Brand With Beans	7.5 oz	345	2

CHIPS

CORN
Health Valley

Health Valley	1 oz	160	0
Health Valley No Salt Added	1 oz	160	0
Health Valley With Cheddar Cheese	1 oz	160	0

POTATO
Health Valley

Country Ripple	1 oz	160	12
Country Ripple No Salt Added	1 oz	160	12
Dip Chips	1 oz	160	12
Dip Chips No Salt Added	1 oz	160	12
Natural	1 oz	160	12
Natural No Salt Added	1 oz	160	12
Kelly's	1 oz	150	3
Kelly's Bar-B-Q	1 oz	150	2

FOOD	PORTION	CAL	VIT E
Kelly's Crunchy	1 oz	150	1
Kelly's Rippled	1 oz	150	3
Kelly's Sour Cream n' Onion	1 oz	150	3
Snyder's	1 oz	150	2
Snyder's Au Gratin	1 oz	150	2
Snyder's BBQ	1 oz	150	2
Snyder's Cajun	1 oz	150	2
Snyder's Coney Island	1 oz	150	2
Snyder's Grilled Steak & Onion	1 oz	150	2
Snyder's Hot Chili	1 oz	150	2
Snyder's Kosher Dill	1 oz	150	2
Snyder's No Salt	1 oz	150	2
Snyder's Salt & Vinegar	1 oz	150	2
Snyder's Smokey Bacon	1 oz	150	2
Snyder's Sour Cream & Onion	1 oz	150	2
Snyder's Sour Cream & Onion, Unsalted	1 oz	150	2
Snyder's Zesty Italian	1 oz	150	2
potato	1 oz	152	1
potato	1 pkg (8 oz)	1217	11
sticks	1 pkg (1 oz)	148	2
sticks	½ cup	94	1

CILANTRO

fresh	¼ cup	1	1

COCOA

Ultra Slim-Fast Hot Cocoa, as prep w/ water	8 oz	190	11

FOOD	PORTION	CAL	VIT E
COCONUT			
fresh	1 piece (1.5 oz)	159	tr
fresh, shredded	1 cup	283	1
COOKIES			
READY-TO-EAT			
Amaranth Cookies (Health Valley)	1	70	4
Fancy Fruit Chunks Apricot Almond (Health Valley)	2	90	2
Fancy Fruit Chunks Date Pecan (Health Valley)	2	90	2
Fancy Fruit Chunks Raisin Oat Bran (Health Valley)	2	70	2
Fancy Fruit Chunks Tropical Fruit (Health Valley)	2	90	11
Fancy Peanut Chunks (Health Valley)	2	90	tr
Fruit & Fitness (Health Valley)	5	200	3
Fruit Jumbos Almond Date (Health Valley)	1	70	1
Fruit Jumbos Raisin Nut (Health Valley)	1	70	1
Fruit Jumbos Tropical Fruit (Health Valley)	1	70	2
Fruit Jumbos Oat Bran (Health Valley)	1	70	1
Graham Amaranth (Health Valley)	7	110	0
Graham Honey (Health Valley)	7	100	6
Graham Oat Bran (Health Valley)	7	120	4
Honey Jumbos Crisp Cinnamon (Health Valley)	1	70	tr
Honey Jumbos Crisp Peanut Butter (Health Valley)	1	70	1
Honey Jumbos Fancy Oat Bran (Health Valley)	2	130	6

FOOD	PORTION	CAL	VIT E
Oat Bran Animal Cookies (Health Valley)	7	110	2
Oat Bran Fruit & Nut (Health Valley)	2	110	1
The Great Tofu (Health Valley)	2	90	tr
The Great Wheat Free (Health Valley)	2	80	tr

CORN

TAKE-OUT

fritters	1 (1 oz)	62	2
scalloped	½ cup	258	1

CORNMEAL

Aunt Jemima White	3 tbsp	102	1
Aunt Jemima Yellow	3 tbsp	102	1
Quaker White	3 tbsp	102	1
Quaker Yellow	3 tbsp	102	1
corn grits, cooked	1 cup	146	tr
corn grits, uncooked	1 cup	579	tr
degermed	1 cup	506	tr
MIX			
Aunt Jemima Bolted White Mix	3 tbsp	99	1
Aunt Jemima Buttermilk Self-Rising White Mix	3 tbsp	101	0
Aunt Jemima Self-Rising White Mix	3 tbsp	98	0

CORNSTARCH

cornstarch	⅛ cup	164	0

CRACKERS

Rice Bran (Health Valley)	7	130	2

CRESS

garden, raw	½ cup	8	tr

FOOD	PORTION	CAL	VIT E
CUCUMBER			
FRESH			
raw	1 (11 oz)	38	tr
raw, sliced	½ cup (1.8 oz)	7	tr
CUSTARD			
zabaglione, home recipe	½ cup (57.2 g)	135	1
DINNER			
FROZEN			
Ultra Slim-Fast Beef Pepper Steak	12 oz	270	2
Ultra Slim-Fast Mesquite Chicken	12 oz	360	3
Ultra Slim-Fast Shrimp Creole	12 oz	240	3
Ultra Slim-Fast Shrimp Marinara	12 oz	290	3
EGG DISHES			
HOME RECIPE			
deviled	2 halves	145	6
TAKE-OUT			
salad	½ cup	307	12
EGG SUBSTITUTES			
Egg Watchers	2 oz	50	1
EGGPLANT			
FRESH			
raw, cut up	½ cup (1.4 oz)	11	tr
whole, peeled, raw	1 (1 lb)	117	tr
FAT			
cocoa butter	1 tbsp	120	tr
lard	1 cup (205 g)	1849	3
lard	1 tbsp (13 g)	115	tr

FOOD	PORTION	CAL	VIT E
FILBERTS			
dried, unblanched	1 oz	179	7
FLOUR			
Self-Rising (Aunt Jemima)	¼ cup	109	0
rye, dark	1 cup	415	2
rye, light	1 cup	374	tr
rye, medium	1 cup	361	tr
triticale whole grain	1 cup	440	tr
white all-purpose	1 cup	455	tr
white cake	1 cup	395	tr
FRENCH TOAST			
FROZEN			
Aunt Jemima	3 oz	166	tr
Aunt Jemima Cinnamon Swirl	3 oz	171	1
FROG'S LEGS			
frog leg, as prep w/ seasoned flour & fried	1 (0.8)	70	0
FRUIT SNACKS			
Health Valley			
Bakes Apple	1 bar	100	3
Bakes Date	1 bar	100	3
Bakes Raisin	1 bar	100	3
Fruit & Fitness Bars	2 bars	200	3
Oat Bran Bakes Apricot	1 bar	100	1
Oat Bran Bakes Fig & Nut	1 bar	110	tr
Oat Bran Jumbo Fruit Bar Almond & Date	1 bar	170	tr
Oat Bran Jumbo Fruit Bars Raisin & Cinnamon	1 bar	160	3

FOOD	PORTION	CAL	VIT E
Rice Bran Jumbo Fruit Bars Almond & Date	1 bar	160	9

GARLIC

clove	1	4	tr

GELATIN

MIX
Jell-O

Apricot	½ cup	82	0
Black Cherry	½ cup	82	0
Black Raspberry	½ cup	82	0
Blackberry	½ cup	82	0
Concord Grape	½ cup	82	0
Lemon	½ cup	82	0
Lime	½ cup	82	0
Mixed Fruit	½ cup	82	0
Orange	½ cup	82	0
Wild Strawberry	½ cup	81	0
low calorie	½ cup	8	0

GRANOLA

BARS

Quaker Chewy Chocolate Chip	1	128	1
Quaker Chewy Chunky Nut & Raisin	1	131	tr
Quaker Chewy Cinnamon Raisin	1	128	1
Quaker Chewy Honey & Oats	1	125	1
Quaker Chewy Peanut Butter	1	128	1
Quaker Chewy Peanut Butter Chocolate Chip	1	131	tr
Quaker Dipps Caramel Nut	1	148	tr
Quaker Dipps Chocolate Chip	1	139	tr

FOOD	PORTION	CAL	VIT E
CEREAL			
Quaker Sun Country 100% Natural With Almonds	¼ cup	130	1
Quaker Sun Country 100% Natural With Raisins & Dates	¼ cup	123	1
Quaker Sun Country With Raisins	¼ cup	125	tr

HAM DISHES

HOME RECIPE			
croquettes	1 (3.1 oz)	217	5
salad	½ cup	287	5

HAMBURGER

TAKE-OUT			
single patty w/ cheese & bun	1 lg	608	1

ICE CREAM AND FROZEN DESSERTS

Ultra Slim-Fast			
Chocolate	4 oz	100	5
Chocolate Fudge	4 oz	120	5
Fudge Bar	1	90	3
Peach	4 oz	100	5
Pralines and Caramel	4 oz	120	5
Vanilla	4 oz	90	5
Vanilla Chocolate Sandwich	1	140	3
Vanilla Cookie Crunch Bar	1	90	3
Vanilla Fudge Cookie	4 oz	110	5
Vanilla Oatmeal Sandwich	1	150	3
Vanilla Sandwich	1	140	3

LAMB DISHES

TAKE-OUT			
curry	¾ cup	345	7

FOOD	PORTION	CAL	VIT E
stew	¾ cup	124	2

LEEKS

FRESH
| raw | 1 (4.4 oz) | 76 | 1 |
| raw, chopped | ¼ cup | 16 | tr |

LENTILS

CANNED
| Health Valley Fast Menu Hearty Lentils Garden Vegetables | 7½ oz | 150 | 1 |

LETTUCE

| iceberg | 1 head (19 oz) | 70 | 2 |
| iceberg | 1 leaf | 3 | tr |

MAYONNAISE

REGULAR
| mayonnaise | 1 cup | 1577 | 69 |
| mayonnaise | 1 tbsp | 99 | 4 |

MILK SUBSTITUTES

Edensoy	8.45 fl oz	140	0
Edensoy Extra	8.45 fl oz	140	8
Vegelicious	8 fl oz	100	3

MUFFIN

FROZEN
Health Valley
Almond & Date Oat Bran Fancy Fruit	1	180	2
Apple Spice Fat Free	1	140	1
Banana Fat Free	1	130	1
Oat Bran Fancy Fruit Blueberry	1	140	3

FOOD	PORTION	CAL	VIT E
Health Valley *(cont.)*			
Oat Bran Fancy Fruit Raisin	1	180	1
Raisin Spice Fat Free	1	140	1
Rice Bran Fancy Fruit Raisin	1	210	4

MUSHROOMS

FRESH
chanterelle	3.5 oz	11	tr
morel	3.5 oz	9	tr
raw	1 (1.5 oz)	5	tr
raw, sliced	½ cup	9	tr

MUSTARD GREENS

raw, chopped	½ cup	7	1

NOODLES

DRY
Egg (Golden Grain)	2 oz	210	0

DRY MIX
Minute Microwave Chicken Flavored	½ cup	157	1
Minute Microwave Parmesan	½ cup	178	1
Ultra Slim-Fast Noodles & Alfredo Sauce	2.3 oz	240	9
Ultra Slim-Fast Noodles & Beef	2.3 oz	230	9
Ultra Slim-Fast Noodles & Cheese	2.3 oz	230	9
Ultra Slim-Fast Noodles & Chicken Sauce	2.3 oz	220	9
Ultra Slim-Fast Noodles & Tomato Herb Sauce	2.3 oz	220	9

TAKE-OUT
noodle pudding	½ cup	132	tr

FOOD	PORTION	CAL	VIT E

NUTRITIONAL SUPPLEMENTS

DIET
Dynatrim

FOOD	PORTION	CAL	VIT E
Dutch Chocolate, as prep w/ 1% milk	8 oz	220	11
Strawberry Royale, as prep w/ 1% milk	8 oz	220	11
Vanilla, as prep w/ 1% milk	8 oz	220	11
Figurines			
Chocolate	1 bar	100	5
Chocolate Caramel	1 bar	100	5
Chocolate Peanut Butter	1 bar	100	5
S'Mores	1 bar	100	5
Vanilla	1 bar	100	5
Slim-Fast			
Nutrition Bar Dutch Chocolate	1	130	11
Nutrition Bar Peanut Butter	1	140	11
Powder Chocolate Malt, as prep w/ skim milk	8 oz	190	11
Powder Chocolate, as prep w/ skim milk	8 oz	190	11
Powder Strawberry, as prep w/ skim milk	8 oz	190	11
Powder Vanilla, as prep w/ skim milk	8 oz	190	11
Ultra Slim-Fast			
Cafe Mocha, as prep w/ skim milk	8 oz	200	11
Chocolate Royale, as prep w/ skim milk	8 oz	200	11
Crunch Bar Cocoa Almond	1	110	5
Crunch Bar Cocoa Raspberry	1	100	5
Crunch Bar Vanilla Almond	1	110	5
Dutch Chocolate, as prep w/ water	8 oz	220	11

FOOD	PORTION	CAL	VIT E
Ultra Slim-Fast *(cont.)*			
French Vanilla, as prep w/ skim milk	8 oz	190	11
French Vanilla, as prep w/ water	8 oz	220	11
Fruit Juice Mix, as prep w/ fruit juice	8 oz	200	11
Pina Colada, as prep w/ skim milk	8 oz	180	11
Ready-to-Drink Chocolate Royale	11 oz	230	11
Ready-to-Drink Chocolate Royale	12 oz	250	11
Ready-to-Drink French Vanilla	11 oz	230	11
Ready-to-Drink French Vanilla	12 oz	220	11
Ready-to-Drink Strawberry Supreme	12 oz	220	11
Strawberry Supreme, as prep w/ water	8 oz	220	11
Strawberry, as prep w/ skim milk	8 oz	190	11

OIL

FOOD	PORTION	CAL	VIT E
Mazola	1 cup	1955	42
Mazola	1 tbsp	120	3
almond	1 cup	1927	128
almond	1 tbsp	120	8
apricot kernel	1 cup	1927	13
apricot kernel	1 tbsp	120	1
coconut	1 tbsp	117	tr
corn	1 cup	1927	47
corn	1 tbsp	120	3
cottonseed	1 cup	1927	115
cottonseed	1 tbsp	120	7
oat	1 tbsp	120	2
olive	1 cup	1909	44

FOOD	PORTION	CAL	VIT E
olive	1 tbsp	119	2
palm	1 cup	1927	63
palm	1 tbsp	120	4
palm kernel	1 cup	1879	8
palm kernel	1 tbsp	117	tr
peanut	1 cup	1909	38
peanut	1 tbsp	119	2
rice bran	1 tbsp	120	7
safflower	1 cup	1927	111
safflower	1 tbsp	120	7
sesame	1 tbsp	120	tr
soybean	1 cup	1927	36
soybean	1 tbsp	120	2
sunflower	1 cup	1927	147
sunflower	1 tbsp	120	9
tomato seed	1 tbsp	120	4
walnut	1 tbsp	120	tr
wheat germ	1 tbsp	120	30

OLIVES

Spanish Green (Tee Pee)	2 oz	98	0

ONION

FROZEN

rings, cooked	2 (0.7 oz)	81	tr

ORIENTAL FOOD

TAKE-OUT

chicken teriyaki	¾	399	12
chop suey w/ pork	1 cup	375	0
chow mein, pork	1 cup	425	10

FOOD	PORTION	CAL	VIT E
chow mein, shrimp	1 cup	221	10
wonton soup	1 cup	205	1
wonton, fried	½ cup (1 oz)	111	7

OYSTERS

stew	1 cup	278	1

PANCAKE/WAFFLE SYRUP

low calorie	1 tbsp	12	0

PANCAKES

FROZEN
Blueberry (Aunt Jemima)	3.48 oz	220	1
Buttermilk (Aunt Jemima)	3.48 oz	210	tr
Buttermilk Batter, as prep (Aunt Jemima)	3.6 oz	180	2
Original (Aunt Jemima)	3.48 oz	211	1
Original Batter, as prep (Aunt Jemima)	3.6 oz	183	1

MIX
Pancake Mix, not prep (Health Valley)	1 oz	100	tr
Whole Wheat Pancake & Waffle Mix (Aunt Jemima)	3 (4-in diam)	270	5

TAKE-OUT
potato	1 (4-in diam)	78	5

PARSLEY

fresh, chopped	½ cup	11	1

PARSNIPS

FRESH
raw, sliced	½ cup	50	1

FOOD	PORTION	CAL	VIT E

PASTA

DRY

FOOD	PORTION	CAL	VIT E
Lasagna, Spinach Whole Wheat (Health Valley)	2 oz	170	12
Lasagna, Whole Wheat (Health Valley)	2 oz	170	tr
Pasta (Golden Grain)	2 oz	203	4
Spaghetti, Amaranth (Health Valley)	2 oz	170	tr
Spaghetti, Spinach Whole Wheat (Health Valley)	2 oz	170	12
Spaghetti, Oat Bran (Health Valley)	2 oz	120	0

PASTA DINNERS

DRY MIX

FOOD	PORTION	CAL	VIT E
Minute Microwave Cheddar Cheese Broccoli and Pasta, as prep	½ cup	160	1
Ultra Slim-Fast Macaroni & Cheese	2.3 oz	230	9

FROZEN

FOOD	PORTION	CAL	VIT E
Ultra Slim-Fast Spaghetti With Beef & Mushroom Sauce	12 oz	370	3

TAKE-OUT

FOOD	PORTION	CAL	VIT E
lasagna	1 piece (2.5×2.5 in)	374	tr
manicotti	¾ cup (6.4 oz)	273	1
rigatoni w/ sausage sauce	¾ cup	260	1
spaghetti w/ meatballs & cheese	1 cup	407	6

PEANUT BUTTER

FOOD	PORTION	CAL	VIT E
Health Valley Chunky No Salt	2 tbsp	170	9
Health Valley Creamy No Salt	2 tbsp	170	9

PEANUTS

FOOD	PORTION	CAL	VIT E
dry roasted	1 cup	855	11
dry roasted	1 oz	164	2

FOOD	PORTION	CAL	VIT E
oil roasted	1 cup	837	10
oil roasted	1 oz	163	2
oil roasted, w/o salt	1 cup	837	10
oil roasted, w/o salt	1 oz	163	2
unroasted	1 oz	159	2

PEAS

FROZEN

green, cooked	½ cup	63	tr

PECANS

dried	1 oz	190	1
halves, dried	1 cup	721	3

PEPPERS

FRESH

green, raw	1 (2.6 oz)	20	1
green, raw, chopped	½ cup	13	tr
red, raw	1 (2.6 oz)	20	1
red, raw, chopped	½ cup	13	tr

PERCH

red, raw	3.5 oz	114	1

PHYLLO DOUGH

Ekizian	½ lb	865	5

PIEROGI

TAKE-OUT

pierogi	¾ cup (4.4 oz)	307	tr

PISTACHIOS

dried	1 cup	739	7

FOOD	PORTION	CAL	VIT E
dried	1 oz	164	1

POPCORN

Ultra Slim-Fast Lite N' Tasty	½ oz	60	3

POTATO

FRESH

baked w/o skin	1 (5 oz)	145	tr
baked w/o skin	½ cup	57	tr
boiled	½ cup	68	tr

PRETZELS

Ultra Slim-Fast Lite N' Tasty	1 oz	100	3

PUDDING

HOME RECIPE

bread w/ raisins	½ cup	180	tr

READY-TO-USE

Butterscotch (Ultra Slim-Fast)	4 oz	100	3
Chocolate (Ultra Slim-Fast)	4 oz	100	3
Vanilla (Ultra Slim-Fast)	4 oz	100	3

TAKE-OUT

rice w/ raisins	½ cup	246	1
tapicoa	½ cup	169	tr

RICE

BROWN

Minute Precooked, as prep	½ cup	121	tr

DRY MIX

Minute Microwave Broccoli Almondine	½ cup	143	tr
Minute Microwave Cheddar Cheese Broccoli	½ cup	164	tr
Minute Microwave French Pilaf	½ cup	133	tr

FOOD	PORTION	CAL	VIT E
Minute Microwave Long Grain Brown And Wild	½ cup	140	tr
Minute Microwave Rice With Savory Cheese Sauce, as prep	½ cup	162	tr
Ultra Slim-Fast Oriental Style	2.3 oz	240	9
Ultra Slim-Fast Rice & Chicken Sauce	2.3 oz	240	9
TAKE-OUT			
pilaf	½ cup	84	tr
spanish	¾ cup	363	tr
WHITE			
long-grain instant, cooked	½ cup	80	tr
long-grain parboiled, cooked	½ cup	100	tr
long-grain, cooked	½ cup	131	tr
short-grain, cooked	½ cup	133	tr

RUTABAGA

FRESH			
cooked, mashed	½ cup	41	tr

SALAD

TAKE-OUT			
chef w/o dressing	1½ cups	386	1
waldorf	½ cup	79	1

SALAD DRESSING

READY-TO-USE			
Ultra Slim-Fast French	1 tbsp	20	2
Ultra Slim-Fast Italian	1 tbsp	6	2

SALMON

TAKE-OUT			
salmon cake	1 (3 oz)	241	1

FOOD	PORTION	CAL	VIT E
SAUCE			
JARRED			
Hot Dog (Wolf Brand)	1.25 oz	44	1
SEAWEED			
FRESH			
kelp	1 oz	12	tr
SEMOLINA			
dry	½ cup	303	tr
SESAME			
seeds, dried	1 cup	825	3
seeds, dried	1 tbsp	52	tr
SHRIMP			
TAKE-OUT			
jambalaya	¾ cup	188	tr
SNACKS			
Cornnuts			
Barbecue	1 oz	120	tr
Nacho Cheese	1 oz	120	tr
Original	1 oz	120	tr
Picante	1 oz	120	tr
Ranch	1 oz	120	tr
Healthy Valley Cheddar Lites	0.75 oz	40	0
Ultra Slim-Fast Lite N' Tasty Cheese Curls	1 oz	110	3
SNAP BEANS			
FRESH			
green, raw	½ cup	17	tr

FOOD	PORTION	CAL	VIT E
FROZEN			
green, cooked	½ cup	18	tr
italian, cooked	½ cup	18	tr
yellow, cooked	½ cup	18	tr

SOUP

CANNED
Health Valley

FOOD	PORTION	CAL	VIT E
Beef Broth	7.5 oz	10	1
Beef Broth No Salt Added	7.5 oz	10	1
Black Bean	7.5 oz	150	6
Black Bean No Salt Added	7.5 oz	150	6
Chicken Broth	7.5 oz	35	tr
Chicken Broth No Salt Added	7.5 oz	35	tr
Chunky Chicken Vegetable	7.5 oz	125	13
Chunky Five Bean Vegetable	7.5 oz	110	tr
Chunky Five Bean Vegetable No Salt Added	7.5 oz	110	tr
Chunky Vegetable Chicken No Salt Added	7.5 oz	125	13
Green Split Pea	7.5 oz	180	tr
Green Split Pea No Salt Added	7.5 oz	180	tr
Lentil	7.5 oz	220	3
Lentil No Salt Added	7.5 oz	220	3
Manhattan Clam Chowder	7.5 oz	110	tr
Manhattan Clam Chowder No Salt Added	7.5 oz	110	tr
Minestrone	7.5 oz	130	tr
Minestrone No Salt Added	7.5 oz	130	tr
Mushroom Barley	7.5 oz	100	5
Mushroom Barley No Salt Added	7.5 oz	100	5
Potato Leek	7.5 oz	130	tr

FOOD	PORTION	CAL	VIT E
Potato Leek No Salt Added	7.5 oz	130	tr
Tomato	7.5 oz	130	5
Tomato No Salt Added	7.5 oz	130	5
Vegetable	7.5 oz	110	5
Vegetable No Salt Added	7.5 oz	110	5
DRY			
Ultra Slim-Fast			
Beef Noodle	6 oz	45	3
Chicken Leek	6 oz	50	3
Chicken Noodle	6 oz	45	3
Creamy Broccoli	6 oz	75	3
Creamy Tomato	6 oz	60	3
Hearty Vegetable	6 oz	50	3
Onion	6 oz	45	3
Potato Leek	6 oz	80	3
HOME RECIPE			
corn & cheese chowder	¾ cup	215	1
greek	¾ cup	63	tr

SPANISH FOOD

FOOD	PORTION	CAL	VIT E
CANNED			
Tamales (Wolf Brand)	7.5 oz	328	2
MIX			
Masa Harina De Maiz (Quaker)	2 tortillas	137	0
Masa Trigo (Quaker)	2 tortillas	149	0

SPINACH

FOOD	PORTION	CAL	VIT E
FRESH			
raw, chopped	½ cup	6	1

STUFFING/DRESSING

FOOD	PORTION	CAL	VIT E
HOME RECIPE			
bread, as prep w/ water egg & fat	½ cup	107	tr

FOOD	PORTION	CAL	VIT E
sausage	½ cup	292	tr
MIX			
Stove Top Chicken, as prep	½ cup	176	tr

SUGAR SUBSTITUTES

S&W Liquid Table Sweetener	⅙ tsp	0	0

TOFU

Mori-Nu Silken Extra-Firm	½ box (5.25 oz)	90	1
Mori-Nu Silken Firm	½ box (5.25 oz)	90	1
Mori-Nu Silken Soft	½ box (5.25 oz)	80	1

TOMATO

CANNED			
Health Valley Sauce	1 cup	70	26
Health Valley Sauce Low Sodium	1 cup	70	26
FRESH			
red	1 (4.5 oz)	26	tr
red, chopped	1 cup	35	1
JUICE			
tomato juice	½ cup	21	tr
tomato juice	6 oz	32	tr

TRITICALE

dry	½ cup	323	2

TUNA

CANNED			
Empress Chunk Light	2 oz	60	1

TURNIPS

FRESH			
cooked, mashed	½ cup (4.2 oz)	47	tr

FOOD	PORTION	CAL	VIT E
cubed, cooked	½ cup (3 oz)	33	tr
greens, raw, chopped	½ cup	7	1

VEAL DISHES

TAKE-OUT

parmigiana	4.2 oz	279	tr

WAFFLES

FROZEN

Apple Cinnamon (Aunt Jemima)	2.5 oz	176	1
Blueberry (Aunt Jemima)	2.5 oz	175	tr
Blueberry Batter, as prep (Aunt Jemima)	3.6 oz	204	tr
Buttermilk (Aunt Jemima)	2.5 oz	179	tr
Original (Aunt Jemima)	2.5 oz	173	tr

WALNUTS

english, dried	1 oz	182	1
english, dried, chopped	1 cup	770	4

WATERCRESS

FRESH

raw, chopped	½ cup	2	tr

WHEAT GERM

Kretschmer	¼ cup	103	10
Kretschmer Honey Crunch	¼ cup	105	8
plaint, toasted	¼ cup	108	6
plain, untoasted	¼ cup	104	6

THE

SUPERMARKET

NUTRITION
COUNTER

**BE A SAVVY SHOPPER WITH
MONEY-SAVING, HEALTH-CONSCIOUS
TIPS FROM TWO NATIONALLY
RECOGNIZED NUTRITION EXPERTS**

OVER 16,000 ITEMS

Annette Natow, Ph.D.,R.D.,
and Jo-Ann Heslin, M.A.,R.D.

**Bestselling Authors of
The Fat Counter and *The Cholesterol Counter***

POCKET
BOOKS

Available from Pocket Books

1076